Boost Immunity

A Comprehensive and Holistic Guide to Boost Immunity

(Discover the Power of Nature to Strengthen Your Body's Defence System)

John Carter

Published By **Phil Dawson**

John Carter

All Rights Reserved

Boost Immunity : A Comprehensive and Holistic Guide to Boost Immunity (Discover the Power of Nature to Strengthen Your Body's Defence System)

ISBN 978-0-9952066-5-6

No part of this guidebook shall be reproduced in any form without permission in writing from the publisher except in the case of brief quotations embodied in critical articles or reviews.

Legal & Disclaimer

The information contained in this book is not designed to replace or take the place of any form of medicine or professional medical advice. The information in this book has been provided for educational & entertainment purposes only.

The information contained in this book has been compiled from sources deemed reliable, and it is accurate to the best of the Author's knowledge; however, the Author cannot guarantee its accuracy and validity and cannot be held liable for any errors or omissions. Changes are periodically made to this book. You must consult your doctor or get professional medical advice before using any of the suggested remedies, techniques, or information in this book.

Upon using the information contained in this book, you agree to hold harmless the Author from and against any damages, costs, and expenses, including any legal fees potentially resulting from the application of any of the information provided by this guide. This disclaimer applies to any damages or injury caused by the use and application, whether directly or indirectly, of any advice or information presented, whether for breach of contract, tort, negligence, personal injury, criminal intent, or under any other cause of action.

You agree to accept all risks of using the information presented inside this book. You need to consult a professional medical practitioner in order to ensure you are both able and healthy enough to participate in this program.

Table Of Contents

Chapter 1: How Does Transcription Paintings? 1

Chapter 2: Dietary Factors 17

Chapter 3: The Importance of a Wholesome Micro Biome 33

Chapter 4: Short-Chain Fatty Acids 45

Chapter 5: Meditation 62

Chapter 6: Additional Assets 85

Chapter 7: Treat Genetic Troubles 100

Chapter 8: Understanding the Immune System 119

Chapter 9: Nourishing Your Body Right. 131

Chapter 10: The Role of Physical Activity 143

Chapter 11: Nature's Gift Sunshine and Fresh Air 160

Chapter 12: Steering Clear of Over-The-Counter Pitfalls 177

Chapter 1: How Does Transcription Paintings?

Transcription starts off evolved at the same time as a protein called RNA polymerase binds to a gene on DNA. RNA polymerase then unwinds the DNA and uses it as a template to make a complementary RNA

Molecule. This RNA molecule is known as messenger RNA (mRNA).

The mRNA molecule is then exported from the nucleus to the cytoplasm, in which it is used as a template for protein synthesis. The process of protein synthesis is referred to as translation.

What are the steps of transcription?

The steps of transcription are:

1. RNA polymerase binds to a gene on DNA.

four. The RNA molecule is exported from the nucleus to the cytoplasm.

Five. The RNA molecule is used as a template for protein synthesis.

What are the goods of transcription?

The merchandise of transcription are:

mRNA: A unmarried-stranded RNA molecule this is complementary to the DNA template strand.

tRNA: A type of RNA molecule that consists of amino acids to the ribosome during protein synthesis.

rRNA: A type of RNA molecule this is a part of the ribosome.

What are the features of transcription?

Transcription is vital for the method of gene expression. It is the first step in the approach through the use of which information from genes is used to make proteins. Transcription is likewise important for the law of gene expression.

What are some problems that have an effect on transcription?

Mutations in genes that encode RNA polymerase can reason troubles together with cystic fibrosis and Duchenne muscular dystrophy. Mutations in genes that encode other proteins worried

in transcription can also motive issues along side fragile X syndrome and Rett syndrome.

Additional sources

[Transcription](

[The basics of transcription]([Transcription and translation](Translation

Translation is the approach with the useful resource of way of which RNA is used to make proteins. It is one of the 3 primary steps of gene expression, along side transcription and splicing. Transcription is the

approach by means of manner of which DNA is copied into RNA, and splicing is the system through which introns (non-coding areas of RNA) are removed from the transcript.

Translation begins offevolved while mRNA binds to a ribosome. The ribosome then reads the mRNA molecule and makes use of it to make a protein. This approach entails the deciphering of the mRNA code into

a sequence of amino acids, which might be the building blocks of proteins.

The mRNA code is examine by way of way of manner of the ribosome in three-base devices referred to as codons. Each codon codes for a selected amino acid. The ribosome moves alongside the mRNA molecule, one codon at a

time, and gives the corresponding amino acid to the developing polypeptide chain. This way continues until the prevent of the mRNA molecule is reached, at which element the polypeptide chain is

released.

Translation is a complicated manner that involves a number of brilliant proteins and RNA molecules. It is important for the producing of proteins, which can be critical for all cell capabilities.

Overview of the Translation Process

The translation way may be divided into 3 main steps:

1.Initiation: The first step in translation is the binding of mRNA to a ribosome. The ribosome is a complex shape composed of protein and RNA molecules. It is responsible

for decoding the mRNA code and assembling the amino acids right into a polypeptide chain.

2.Elongation: Once the mRNA is effective to the ribosome, the elongation segment begins. During this phase, the ribosome moves alongside the mRNA molecule, one codon at a time. As the

ribosome actions, it offers the corresponding amino acid to the growing polypeptide chain.

three.Termination: The termination phase of translation takes place even as the ribosome reaches a prevent codon. A forestall codon is a three-base collection that indicators the quit of the

translation procedure. When the ribosome reaches a save you codon, it releases the polypeptide chain and the translation gadget is complete.

The Genetic Code

The genetic code is the set of rules that govern how the mRNA code is translated proper into a polypeptide chain. The genetic code is a triplet code, because of this that that every codon consists

of 3 bases. Each codon codes for a selected amino acid. The genetic code is time-venerated, due to this that it's far the equal in all organisms.

The Ribosome

The ribosome is a complex form composed of protein and RNA molecules. It is liable for deciphering the mRNA code and assembling the amino acids right right right into a three-dimensional form, which determines its function.Translation Disorders

Translation issues are a hard and fast of genetic issues which can be because of mutations within the genes that encode for the proteins worried in translation. These problems can reason

quite some symptoms, together with developmental delay, highbrow incapacity, and speech and language issues.

Translation is a complex technique that is critical for the production of proteins. It is a testomony to the tremendous complexity of the human body that this method can occur with such precision and accuracy.

Post-translational amendment

Post-translational alternate (PTM) is the manner through which proteins are similarly changed after they may be made. This can contain the addition of chemical companies, the removal of chemical companies, or the folding of the protein into its very last form. PTM is vital for the right function of proteins, and it is able to additionally be used to modify their hobby.

There are many precise sorts of PTMs, and that they can be categorised in keeping with the chemical institution that is brought or eliminated. Some of the maximum not unusual PTMs encompass:

Phosphorylation, which entails the addition of a phosphate organization to the protein. Phosphorylation is a common manner to spark off or deactivate proteins.

Acetylation, which includes the addition of an acetyl business enterprise to the protein. Acetylation will have an effect on the stableness of the protein, further to its ability to bind to distinct proteins.

Methylation, which incorporates the addition of a methyl group to the protein. Methylation can also have an effect on the stability of the protein, as well as its capability to bind to at least one-of-a-type proteins.

Ubiquitination, which entails the addition of a ubiquitin molecule to the protein. Ubiquitination is an indication that the protein is to be degraded.

PTMs moreover may be categorized consistent with wherein they stand up on the protein. Some of the maximum commonplace websites of PTM encompass:

The N-terminus, this is the amino acid at the beginning of the protein.The C-terminus, which is the amino acid on the give up of the protein.The facet chains of amino acids.

PTMs may have a huge effect at the feature of proteins. For instance, regulated.

Functions of PTMs

PTMs serve an entire lot of abilities, which incorporates:

Stabilizing proteins. PTMs can help to stabilize proteins through manner of stopping them from being degraded with the useful resource of enzymes.

Activating or deactivating proteins. PTMs can change the pastime of proteins via altering their shape or their capability to bind to different proteins.

Regulating the interest of proteins. PTMs may be used to adjust the interest of proteins by using way of controlling their expression, their localization, or their interactions with specific proteins.

Marking proteins for degradation. PTMs may be used to mark proteins for degradation thru enzymes.

Mechanisms of PTMs

PTMs can be catalyzed via numerous enzymes, at the side of:

Protein kinases, which catalyze the addition of phosphate companies to proteins. Acetylases, which catalyze the addition of acetyl agencies to proteins. Methyltransferases, which catalyze the addition of methyl organizations to proteins. Ubiquitin ligases, which catalyze the addition of ubiquitin molecules to

proteins.

The particular mechanism of PTMs can variety relying on the sort of PTM and the enzyme that catalyzes it. However, all PTMs contain the switch of a chemical corporation from one molecule to a few exceptional.

Applications of PTMs

PTMs are important for the proper characteristic of proteins. However, PTMs can also be used to manipulate the feature of proteins for recuperation functions. For instance, PTMs can be

used to:

Activate or deactivate proteins. PEnvironmental elements

The surroundings in which a cell lives will have an effect on gene expression. For example, publicity to pollutants or toxins can harm DNA and bring about changes in gene expression.DNA harm

DNA harm may be because of a number of environmental elements, at the side of:

Chemicals: Some chemical substances, along with benzene and formaldehyde, can damage DNA through way of forming covalent bonds with DNA bases. This can result in mutations, which are changes within the

DNA collection.

Radiation: Exposure to radiation, together with UV mild or X-rays, can harm

DNA with the aid of breaking the DNA spine. This can also reason mutations.

Viruses: Some viruses, together with the human papillomavirus (HPV), can insert

their DNA into the DNA of quite a number cell. This can result in mutations and most cancers.

Changes in gene expression

DNA damage can reason changes in gene expression. This is because of the reality DNA harm can prevent genes from being transcribed into mRNA, that is the molecule this is used to make

proteins. If a gene isn't transcribed, then the protein that it codes for will no longer be produced.

Changes in gene expression have to have an entire lot of results on the cell, which include:

Altered cell increase: Changes in gene expression can result in out of control cellular boom, that may reason maximum cancers.

Altered metabolism: Changes in gene expression can reason changes within the manner that the cell uses nutrients, that could bring about a number of fitness issues.

Altered immune feature: Changes in gene expression can bring about impaired immune characteristic, that could make the frame extra at risk of infection.

Environmental elements also can have an effect on gene expression via changing epigenetics

Epigenetics is the take a look at of the manner environmental factors may want to have an effect on gene expression with out converting the DNA series. Epigenetic adjustments are frequently because of chemical adjustments

Chapter 2: Dietary Factors

The meals which you devour can have an effect on gene expression. For instance, consuming a weight loss program rich in fruits and vegetables has been validated to sell healthful gene expression. Conversely, consuming a

eating regimen high in processed components and perilous fats can cause adjustments in gene expression that boom the danger of chronic illnesses together with heart ailment, most cancers, and diabetes.

How do nutritional elements have an effect on gene expression?

Dietary factors could have an impact on gene expression in some of techniques. For instance, nice vitamins can bind to receptors at the surface of cells and spark off signaling pathways that bring about changes in gene expression. Other nutrients can have an effect on gene expression through altering the ranges of hormones and unique molecules that modify gene pastime.

What are the consequences of dietary factors on gene expression?

The effects of nutritional factors on gene expression are complicated and vary relying at the particular nutrient, the dose, and the person. However, some fashionable developments had been located. For instance, consuming a diet rich in give up end result and greens has been established to sell healthful gene expression, at the same time as eating a diet plan immoderate in processed substances and bad fats can lead

to adjustments in gene expression that increase the risk of continual illnesses.

How can you operate dietary factors to sell healthful gene expression?

There are a number of techniques that you may use dietary elements to promote healthy gene expression. Some of the most critical encompass:

Eating a diet plan rich in end end result and veggies. Fruits and vegetables are entire of nutrients, minerals, and exceptional nutrients which may be essential for healthy gene expression.

Limiting your intake of processed materials and perilous fats. Processed ingredients and lousy fats are frequently excessive in strength and coffee in vitamins, and they could make contributions to infection and other health troubles that may purpose modifications in gene expression.

Eating loads of whole grains. Whole grains are a outstanding supply of fiber, vitamins, minerals, and special vitamins which might be crucial for wholesome gene expression.

Choosing lean protein property. Lean protein assets, collectively with fish, chook, andLifestyle factors

Your manner of lifestyles choices can also have an impact on gene expression. For instance, smoking, consuming alcohol, and being obese can all result in modifications in gene expression.

Smoking

Smoking is one of the maximum nicely-studied lifestyle factors that might have an effect on gene expression. Cigarette smoke includes lots of chemical substances, lots of which may be mentioned to be risky

to cells. These chemical materials can harm DNA and bring about changes in gene expression. For example, smoking has been verified to growth the expression of genes which can be concerned in inflammation

and maximum cancers.

Drinking alcohol

Drinking alcohol also can have an effect on gene expression. Alcohol can harm DNA and bring about modifications in the expression of genes which can be worried in mobile increase and differentiation. For

instance, alcohol has been tested to growth the expression of genes which may be involved in most cancers.

Being overweight or obese

Being overweight or overweight is every different life-style element that could have an impact on gene expression. Excess body fat can result in contamination, that could harm DNA and result in changes in gene expression. For example, being obese or obese has been proven to increase the expression of genes which can be concerned in insulin resistance and diabetes.

Other lifestyle elements

Other life-style factors that could have an impact on gene expression encompass diet plan, exercising, and strain. A healthful diet, ordinary workout, and suitable stress manage can all assist to sell

wholesome gene expression.

Your way of life alternatives may have a large impact for your fitness. By making healthful options, you could help to shield your genes and sell proper health.[Drinking Alcohol and Gene Expression](

[Being Overweight or Obese and Gene Expression]([Other Lifestyle Factors and Gene Expression](Introduction

Gene expression is the approach by means of way of which genes are became proteins. Proteins are the building blocks of our our our our bodies and are responsible for everything from our hair coloration to our immune tool. By expertise how gene expression works, we are capable of learn how to hack our genes and beautify our fitness and well-being.

What is Gene Expression?

Gene expression is the way through which records encoded in DNA is transformed right into a practical product, which encompass a protein. This method takes vicinity in steps: transcription and

translation.

Transcription is the device through manner of which DNA is copied into RNA. RNA is a unmarried-stranded molecule this is similar to DNA, however it consists of the sugar ribose in preference to deoxyribose. During transcription, a gene is copied from DNA into RNA through manner of an enzyme called RNA polymerase.

Translation is the method via way of which RNA is transformed proper into a protein. This manner takes vicinity in the ribosome, a small organelle observed in the cytoplasm of cells. During translation, the RNA collection is take a look at through the ribosome and the corresponding amino acids are assembled proper into a protein.

How Does Gene Expression Work?

The approach of gene expression is complex and tightly regulated. In order for a gene to be expressed, a number of steps ought to occur within the proper order. These steps encompass:

DNA methylation. DNA methylation is a chemical modification that takes place on the DNA molecule. It can both silence or spark off genes.

Histone change. Histones are proteins that wrap spherical DNA and help to prepare it into chromosomes. Histone trade also can have an impact on gene expression.

Chromosome form. The way that chromosomes are prepared can have an impact on gene expression. For instance, genes which is probably placed near together on a chromosome are more likely

to be expressed together.

Transcription factors. Transcription factors are proteins that bind to DNA and adjust transcription. They can each spark off or inhibit transcription of a gene.

RNA splicing. RNA splicing is the way via using which introns (non-coding regions of RNA) are eliminated and exons (coding areas of RNA) are joined collectively. This

Gene expression is crucial for life. It is the method by which our our bodies create the proteins that we need to function. Proteins are answerable for everything from our hair shade to our immune device. By knowledge how gene expression works, we are able to discover ways to hack our genes and enhance our health and properly-being.

Here are a few examples of procedures gene expression can be hacked to decorate health and nicely-being:

Gene therapy. Gene treatment is a remedy that consists of placing a practical gene into a affected man or woman's cells to update a defective gene. This may be used to treat loads of genetic sicknesses, which consist of cystic fibrosis and sickle cell anemia.

CRISPR-Cas9 gene editing. CRISPR-Cas9 is a gene-improving device that allows scientists to make unique changes to DNA. This generation has the capability to be used to deal with a

large kind of ailments, which include maximum cancers and HIV.

Nutrition and exercise. Our food regimen and exercising behavior will have an effect on gene expression. For instance, ingesting a wholesome diet and exercising frequently can assist to promote healthy gene

expression and decrease the danger of sickness.

Stress manipulate. Stress can also have an impact on gene expression. Chronic pressure can result in modifications in gene expression which can boom the danger of illness. Conversely, stress

manipulate strategies can assist to promote healthful gene expression and

How to Hack Your Genes

Your genes play a superb position in determining your health and nicely-being. However, your genes are not set in stone. They may be precipitated via your environment, your way of lifestyles, and

your selections. This method that you could honestly "hack" your genes and decorate your fitness and properly-being.

Here are some hints for hacking your genes:

Eat a wholesome weight loss plan. Eating a weight loss plan rich in give up result, vegetables, and entire grains has been showed to promote wholesome gene expression. These ingredients consist of antioxidants and one-of-a-type

vitamins that would assist to protect your DNA from harm. They moreover incorporate fiber, that could help to regulate your blood sugar degrees and decrease infection.

Exercise often. Exercise has been tested to enhance gene expression thru decreasing infection and strain. Exercise moreover allows to beautify your cardiovascular health and

lessen your chance of continual illnesses.

Additional tips:

Take dietary supplements. There are a number of supplements that may help to sell wholesome gene expression. Some of the pleasant supplements encompass:

Green tea extract

Omega-three fatty acids

Get everyday checkups. Your physician can help you to apprehend any genetic dangers that you can have. They also can suggest techniques to reduce your hazard of growing chronic

illnesses.

Talk to a genetic counselor. A genetic counselor will will let you to apprehend your genetic dangers and the manner they may have an impact in your health. They additionally assist you to to make informed

alternatives approximately your health care.

Hacking your genes is not a short restoration. It takes time and effort to make modifications to your way of life. However, the blessings are surely nicely really worth it. By following these suggestions, you can beautify

your health and well-being and reduce your danger of developing continual ailments.

Here are a few extra assets that you may locate useful:

[The National Human Genome Research Institute]([The Genetic Literacy Project]

Gene expression is the technique via which our genes are became proteins. These proteins then control our cells and our bodies. By knowledge how gene expression works, we

can learn how to hack our genes and enhance our fitness and properly-being.

Here are a number of the techniques that we can hack our genes:

We can use gene remedy to correct genetic defects. This includes putting a healthy replica of a gene right into a cell that is missing or has a faulty reproduction of the gene. Gene remedy has been used to address masses of illnesses, including cystic fibrosis, sickle mobile anemia, and HIV.

We can use epigenetics to exchange the manner that genes are expressed. Epigenetics is the check of approaches environmental elements can flip genes on and stale. By revolutionize the manner that we address ailments and decorate our fitness and well-being.

Chapter 3: The Importance of a Wholesome Micro Biome

A healthful microbiome is essential for preserving a healthy weight and stopping persistent sicknesses which includes weight issues and diabetes. A wholesome microbiome permits to alter your urge for food and metabolism, and it could additionally assist to prevent the development of infection, this is a first-rate chance factor for persistent illnesses.

If you're obese or obese, you're much more likely to have an dangerous microbiome. This is because of the truth the dangerous diet plan that is regularly associated with obesity can reason modifications

Eating a healthful diet plan this is wealthy in end result, greens, and entire grains.Limiting your intake of processed meals, sugary drinks, and dangerous fat.Getting regular workout.

Managing strain ranges.

Probiotics are live microorganisms that might assist to enhance your microbiome.

They are available in supplements and in some fermented components, together with yogurt and kefir.

By following these hints, you can help to beautify your microbiome and promote digestive health.

The microbiome performs a essential function in digesting food and maintaining a wholesome weight. By eating a wholesome weight-reduction plan, getting normal workout, and coping with stress stages, you may help

to beautify your microbiome and sell digestive fitness.

How the microbiome protects you from ailment

The microbiome is the community of trillions of micro organism, viruses, fungi, and special microorganisms that live in and to your body. These microorganisms play a vital position in your

fitness by means of using using helping to digest meals, produce nutrients, and combat off infections.

One of the techniques that the microbiome lets in to shield you from illness is through producing antimicrobial materials that kill dangerous bacteria. These substances include bacteriocins,

which might be proteins that inhibit the boom of various micro organism, and defensins, which might be small peptides that kill bacteria via way of way of destructive their cellular walls.

The microbiome additionally allows to adjust your immune tool, that is responsible for stopping off infections. The immune tool is crafted from a community of cells, tissues, and organs

that paintings together to guard you from disease. The microbiome enables to regulate the immune gadget via presenting it with statistics about the surroundings and with the aid of manufacturing molecules that

promote tolerance to harmless bacteria.

A wholesome microbiome is vital for preserving a sturdy immune system and preventing illness. When the microbiome is out of stability, it could result in some of health issues,

including infections, hypersensitive reactions, and autoimmune illnesses.

Here are some of the approaches that a healthy microbiome can help to guard you from

Helps to digest food. The microbiome allows to digest meals with the useful aid of producing enzymes that damage down carbohydrates, proteins, and fat.

Produces vitamins. The microbiome produces some of vitamins, which includes eating regimen B12, vitamins K, and folate.

Protects towards hypersensitive reactions and autoimmune sicknesses. The microbiome lets in to defend towards allergies and autoimmune illnesses via way of the use of regulating the immune device.

A healthful microbiome is essential for preserving a sturdy immune device and preventing sickness. By ingesting a healthy food regimen, getting sufficient workout, and reducing stress, you could

assist to maintain your microbiome in stability and defend yourself from disease.

References

How the microbiome regulates your immune device

The microbiome is the community of trillions of bacteria, viruses, fungi, and notable microorganisms that stay in and on our our our our bodies. These microbes play a vital feature in our fitness

with the aid of the use of supporting us digest food, combat off infections, and modify our immune gadget.

The immune device is a complex network of cells, tissues, and organs that paintings together to guard us from risky micro organism, viruses, and one in all a kind threats. The microbiome plays a key

feature in regulating the immune tool via way of way of manufacturing molecules that talk with immune cells and help to preserve them in stability.

When the microbiome is wholesome, it facilitates to hold the immune device in test, stopping it from overreacting to harmless substances and causing allergic reactions or allergic reactions. However, at the same time as

the microbiome is disrupted, it could bring about an overactive immune device that could reason persistent illnesses together with inflammatory bowel contamination, more than one sclerosis, and rheumatoid arthritis.

Research is increasingly displaying that the microbiome plays a crucial feature in regulating our immune device and that preserving a healthful microbiome is essential for suitable fitness.

Here are some of the strategies that the microbiome regulates the immune system:

Producing antimicrobial compounds. The microbiome produces quite some

A wholesome microbiome is essential for preserving a sturdy immune system and stopping continual ailments. By ingesting a wholesome healthy eating plan, getting sufficient workout, and lowering pressure,

you can assist to keep your microbiome healthful and promote specific fitness.

Here are a few pointers for maintaining a healthy microbiome:

Eat a healthy eating plan rich in end result, veggies, and entire grains.

Avoid processed components, sugary beverages, and awful fats.

Get everyday exercise.

Reduce pressure.

Get enough sleep.

Probiotics and prebiotics can also help to promote a healthy microbiome.How the microbiome synthesizes vitamins and different nutrients

The human frame is home to trillions of bacteria, viruses, and exceptional microorganisms, together referred to as the microbiome. These microbes play a essential feature in our health, assisting

us to digest food, fight off infections, and bring crucial nutrients.

One of the most essential abilties of the microbiome is to synthesize nutrients and amazing vitamins that our our our bodies can't produce on their non-public. These encompass vitamins B12, K, and

folate, in addition to short-chain fatty acids (SCFAs).

Vitamin B12

Vitamin B12 is a water-soluble weight-reduction plan this is vital for a healthful worried system. It is also involved inside the production of crimson blood cells and DNA.

Most people get their food regimen B12 from animal products, which include meat, fish, and dairy products. However, some humans, consisting of vegans and vegetarians, might not get sufficient vitamins

B12 from their weight loss plan.

The proper facts is that the microbiome can produce nutrition B12. In truth, some studies have established that humans with a healthy microbiome have higher ranges of vitamins B12 than humans

with a less wholesome microbiome.

Vitamin K

Vitamin K is a fats-soluble vitamins this is important for blood clotting. It is also Most people get their nutrition K from inexperienced leafy greens, which consist of spinach, kale, and broccoli. However, some human beings won't get sufficient eating regimen K from their healthy dietweight-reduction plan.

The microbiome also can produce nutrients K. In reality, one have a have a look at located that humans with a wholesome microbiome had better tiers of nutrients K of their blood than human beings with a miles tons less

healthful microbiome.

Folate, moreover referred to as food plan B9, is a water-soluble weight loss plan this is important for a healthy pregnancy. It is likewise involved in the manufacturing of pink blood cells and DNA.

Most humans get their folate from give up stop end result, veggies, and complete grains. However, a few humans, collectively with pregnant ladies and people with sure scientific situations, also can want to take a

folate complement.

The microbiome also can produce folate. In truth, one have a look at determined that people with a wholesome microbiome had higher stages of folate in their blood than human beings with a far tons much less healthful

microbiome.

Chapter 4: Short-Chain Fatty Acids

Short-chain fatty acids (SCFAs) are a kind of fatty acid that is produced with the useful useful resource of the fermentation of fiber inside the colon. SCFAs have some of health advantages, on the aspect of enhancing

digestion, reducing inflammation, and boosting immunity.

The microbiome is responsible for the manufacturing of SCFAs. In fact, one have a take a look at placed that human beings with a healthful microbiome had better degrees of SCFAs of their stool than people

with a far much less healthy microbiome.

The microbiome performs a critical position in the synthesis of nutrients and other vitamins. By maintaining a healthy microbiome, we're able to help to ensure that we get the nutrients we need to live healthful.

Here are some tips for maintaining a healthful microbiome:Get sufficient sleep.

Manage stress.

Take probiotics and prebiotics.

By following those tips, you may assist to maintain your microbiome wholesome and make sure that you get the nutrients you need to stay wholesome.

How the microbiome influences your mood and conduct

The microbiome is the community of trillions of micro organism, viruses, and other microorganisms that live in and to your frame. These microbes play a crucial position for your health, with the aid of

helping you digest food, fight off infections, and alter your immune tool. They moreover produce neurotransmitters, that are chemical materials that talk among nerve cells. These

neurotransmitters can have an effect to your mood, behavior, and sleep patterns.

How the microbiome affects your temper

The microbiome has been shown to have an impact for your mood in a number of techniques. For example, studies have located that people with despair and tension have a propensity to have precise microbiomes

than individuals who aren't depressed or disturbing. In one observe, humans with despair were found to have lower ranges of Lactobacillus, a kind of micro organism that has been validated to deliver

serotonin, a neurotransmitter that is involved in temper law. Other research have decided that human beings with anxiety generally have a tendency to have better tiers of the bacteria Enterococcus faecalis, which

has been connected to infection and pressure.

How the microbiome influences your behavior

The microbiome can also have an impact to your behavior. For example, studies have determined that human beings with autism spectrum disorder tend to have one-of-a-kind microbiomes than those who do no longer

have autism. In one have a study, youngsters with autism had been observed to have decrease stages of Bifidobacterium, a shape of micro organism that has been established to promote social conduct. Other studies have determined that people with schizophrenia have a tendency to have higher tiers of the micro organism Clostridium difficile, which has been associated with aggression and violence.

How the microbiome affects your sleep patterns

The microbiome also can have an impact on your sleep patterns. For instance, research have retaining a wholesome mood and conduct. By consuming a healthful healthy eating plan, getting enough workout, and decreasing pressure, you could assist to keep your microbiome healthy and beautify your temper,

conduct, and sleep patterns.

Here are a few recommendations for keeping a healthful microbiome:

Eat a healthy dietweight-reduction plan wealthy in fruits, greens, and complete grains.

Avoid processed food, sugary beverages, and excessive quantities of red meat.Get regular exercise.

Reduce stress.

Take probiotics and prebiotics.

Probiotics are live microorganisms that may be decided in meals together with yogurt, kefir, and sauerkraut. They can assist to decorate your gut fitness and boom your immune device.

Prebiotics are non-digestible carbohydrates that feed the probiotics for your gut. You can discover prebiotics in factors at the side of onions, garlic, and asparagus.

By following those guidelines, you can assist to maintain your microbiome wholesome and beautify your mood, behavior, and sleep styles.

Eating a Healthy Diet

Eating a healthy diet is one of the terrific techniques to beautify your simple fitness and properly-being. A healthy healthy dietweight-reduction plan is rich in end result, vegetables, and whole grains, and it limits bad fat, processed elements, and brought sugar. Eating a wholesome healthy dietweight-reduction plan allow you to hold a healthful weight, reduce your chance of chronic ailments like heart illness, stroke, kind 2

diabetes, and some types of maximum cancers, and improve your temper and strength stages.

What is a healthful food plan?

A healthful diet is one which gives your body with the nutrients it desires to characteristic nicely. These vitamins embody carbohydrates, proteins, fats, vitamins, and minerals. Carbohydrates are your frame's most essential supply of electricity, and they arrive from elements like end result, veggies, and grains. Proteins are crucial for building and repairing tissues, and they come

from meals like meat, hen, fish, beans, and nuts. Fats are also critical in your body, and they come from substances like oils, nuts, and seeds. Vitamins and minerals are important for a

style of physical abilties, and they arrive from pretty some additives.

How to consume a wholesome dietChoose entire grains over diffused grains.

Choose lean protein assets.

Limit lousy fats, processed elements, and brought sugar.Drink masses of water.

If you are not certain the manner to eat a healthy food regimen, there are various assets available that will help you. Your scientific doctor or a registered dietitian can offer you with customized recommendation. You

also can discover many useful assets online.

Benefits of ingesting a healthful healthy eating plan

Eating a healthful diet plan has many advantages to your standard fitness and properly-being. These blessings embody:

Improved digestion. A healthy healthy dietweight-reduction plan can help to enhance your digestion via using manner of supplying your frame with the vitamins it wants to deliver digestive enzymes and acids. Eating a wholesome weight-reduction plan also can help to lessen contamination within the digestive tract, that would decorate signs and signs and symptoms of conditions like irritable bowel syndrome (IBS).

Reduced contamination. Eating a healthful weight loss plan can assist to lessen inflammation within the direction of your body. This is because of the fact a healthy weight loss plan is rich in antioxidants, which assist to

defend cells from harm. Inflammation is associated with a number of continual ailments, so lowering contamination can help to reduce your risk of those ailments.

Increased immunity. A healthful weight loss plan can assist to enhance your immune machine. This is due to the fact a healthy weight loss plan is wealthy in vitamins and minerals, which is probably crucial for a healthful immune device. Eating a wholesome healthy eating plan can also help to lessen contamination, which can help to beautify your immune feature.

Better mood. A healthful weight loss program can help to beautify your temper. This is due to the fact a wholesome healthy eating plan is wealthy in nutrients which is probably important for mind characteristic. Eating a healthy diet regime also can assist to reduce contamination, that could enhance your temper.

Reduced threat of continual illnesses. Eating a wholesome weight loss plan can assist to lessen your risk of continual diseases like coronary heart sickness, stroke, kind 2 diabetes, and some styles of most cancers. This is due to the fact a healthy diet plan is wealthy in vitamins which can be crucial for a wholesome coronary coronary coronary heart, mind, and immune device. Eating a healthy weight-reduction plan can also help to reduce contamination,

this is associated with some of chronic illnesses.

Conclusion

Eating a healthy food plan is one of the satisfactory strategies to beautify your typical health andHow workout benefits your microbiome

Increases blood glide to the intestines. Exercise will boom blood float to all components of the body, which consist of the intestines. This expanded blood go along with the waft permits to enhance the absorption of nutrients and the increase of useful micro organism.

Reduces stress. Exercise has been demonstrated to lessen stress tiers. Stress may be dangerous to the microbiome, as it could reason contamination and the growth of risky micro organism.

Boosts immunity. Exercise has been shown to beautify immunity. A healthful immune machine is critical for preserving a wholesome microbiome.

Improves mood. Exercise has been proven to decorate temper. A precise temper is associated with a healthful microbiome.

Specific sorts of exercise which is probably accurate in your microbiome

Walking is a tremendous way to get started out out out with workout. It is simple on the joints and may be accomplished at any time of day.

Running is a extra extreme form of exercise than on foot. It is a exquisite manner to burn electricity and improve your cardiovascular fitness.

Cycling is a amazing manner to get some workout and explore your environment. It is likewise a notable manner to alleviate strain.

Swimming is a first rate manner to get workout and cool off on a warmth day. It is also a low-impact interest that is straightforward at the joints.

Yoga andPilates are excellent methods to enhance your flexibility and center electricity. They also are acceptable for decreasing strain.

How plenty exercising do you need?

The amount of exercise you want to get to enhance your microbiome relies upon for your person fitness level and desires. However, maximum adults need to cause for at least a hundred and fifty mins of mild-depth cardio hobby or 75 minutes of active-intensity cardio interest every week.

Getting commenced out with workout

If you are new to workout, start slowly and step by step increase the quantity of time and intensity of your workout routines over time. It is likewise essential to concentrate in your body and rest while you want to.

Talk in your physician

Stress is a primary trouble which can negatively impact the microbiome. When you are careworn, your body produces hormones that might harm the useful bacteria on your intestine. Stress

also can bring about risky ingesting behavior, that could further make a contribution to microbiome imbalances.

Symptoms of strain

The signs and signs and symptoms of pressure can range from individual to character, however some common signs and signs and symptoms embody:

Feeling annoying or on area

Having hassle sound asleep

Feeling irritable or moody

Having trouble concentrating

Experiencing bodily signs and signs and symptoms together with complications, stomachaches, or muscle

aches

Having modifications in urge for food or weightAvoiding social sports

How stress affects the micro biome

When you're forced, your frame produces hormones including cortisol and adrenaline. These hormones can damage the useful micro organism to your gut, that would result in a number of

health issues. For instance, studies has confirmed that stress can boom the risk of growing weight problems, diabetes, and coronary coronary heart sickness.

Stress can also result in risky ingesting conduct, together with eating extra junk meals or skipping meals. This can in addition make a contribution to microbiome imbalances.

Ways to reduce strain

There are quite a few of factors you could do to reduce strain, inclusive of:

Mindfulness

Spending time in nature

Spending time with loved onesGetting sufficient sleep

Chapter 5: Meditation

Meditation is a exercising that involves focusing in your breath or a selected object if you want to accumulate a country of rest. Meditation has been established to be effective in lowering strain, anxiety, and despair.

Yoga is a mind-frame exercise that combines bodily postures, respiratory bodily activities, and meditation. Yoga has been tested to be effective in reducing strain, anxiety, and depression.

Mindfulness

Mindfulness is a exercise that involves being attentive to the existing 2nd, without judgment. Mindfulness has been shown to be powerful in lowering strain, tension, and

depression.

Spending time in nature

Spending time in nature has been proven to have some of advantages for intellectual fitness, which includes lowering stress, tension, and depression.

Spending time with cherished ones

Spending time with cherished ones can assist to reduce stress and beautify your mood.

Getting enough sleep

Getting enough sleep is crucial for preferred health and nicely-being. When you're sleep-deprived, your body produces greater pressure hormones, that may motive prolonged pressure

degrees.

By reducing stress, you may assist to beautify your common health and nicely-being, and you could additionally help to create a extra healthy microbiome.

Getting Enough Sleep

Getting sufficient sleep is a few different vital way to hack your microbiome. When you are sleep-disadvantaged, your body produces hormones that might damage the beneficial bacteria for your

How sleep influences your microbiome

When you sleep, your frame goes thru a manner referred to ascircadian rhythm. This is a herbal cycle that regulates your sleep-wake cycle and other physical abilties. During

sleep, your frame produces hormones that assist to restore and repair your cells, collectively with the cells in your intestine. These hormones moreover help to regulate your immune tool and metabolism.

When you're sleep-disadvantaged, your frame's circadian rhythm is disrupted. This can motive a number of troubles, which include:

Increased irritation: When you're sleep-deprived, your body produces greater of the pressure hormone cortisol. This can bring about irritation, that could harm the useful

bacteria in your gut.

Altered immune characteristic: Sleep deprivation also can purpose impaired immune feature. This must make you extra liable to infection and infection.

Unhealthy consuming conduct: When you are sleep-disadvantaged, you are more likely to make risky meals picks. This can result in weight advantage and special fitness problems.

Tips for purchasing a tremendous night time time's sleep

There are a number of of things you may do to decorate your sleep conduct and get an great night time's sleep. These embody:

Go to mattress and wake up at the same time every day, even on weekends. This will assist to alter your circadian rhythm and make it easier to fall asleep at night.

Create a calming bedtime routine. This can also need to encompass taking a warmness bath, analyzing a ebook, or taking note of calming music.

Avoid caffeine and alcohol in advance than mattress. These materials can intervene with sleep.

Make sure your bed room is dark, quiet, and funky. These situations are pleasant for sleep.

Getting enough sleep is critical on your usual health and nicely-being. By following those suggestions, you can decorate your sleep habits and get an awesome night time's sleep, on the manner to help

to enhance your microbiome and famous fitness.

Avoiding Harmful Chemicals and Toxins

off incredible micro organism and promoting the growth of awful bacteria.

Pesticides: Pesticides are used to kill pests, however additionally they may be dangerous to human beings. Pesticides can input the body thru the pores and skin, lungs, or digestive tract, and might harm the microbiome by killing off proper bacteria.

Household cleaners: Household cleaners encompass quite some chemical substances that may be unstable to the microbiome. These chemical compounds can input the frame through the pores and pores and skin, lungs, or digestive tract, and may damage the microbiome via killing off authentic micro organism.

Personal care merchandise: Personal care products, which include shampoos, conditioners, and creams, incorporate plenty of chemical materials that can be volatile to the microbiome. These

chemical compounds can enter the body via the pores and pores and pores and skin, and can damage the microbiome with the aid of manner of killing off correct bacteria.

Food additives: Food additives are added to meals to enhance their taste, coloration, or texture. However, some meals additives may be risky to the microbiome. These chemical materials

can enter the body thru the digestive tract, and might harm the microbiome through using killing off real bacteria.

By fending off publicity to these risky chemical substances and pollutants, you can help to defend your microbiome and enhance your normal fitness. Here are some suggestions for maintaining off publicity to

risky chemical substances and pollutants:

Reduce your exposure to air pollutants via using the use of heading off closely polluted areas, strolling or cycling rather than the usage of, and the usage of public transportation at the same time as possible.

Quit smoking or keep away from publicity to secondhand smoke.

Use natural produce each time viable.

Wash your stop result and veggies very well earlier than consuming them.

Choose cleansing merchandise which might be freed from harmful chemical compounds.

Use herbal personal care products, which incorporates shampoos, conditioners, and lotions which are made with plant-primarily based completely factors.

Eat a diet wealthy in end result, vegetables, and whole grains.

Take probiotics and/or prebiotics to assist useful useful resource the boom of right bacteria within the microbiome.

By following those recommendations, you can help to defend your microbiome and enhance your famous health.

Additional tips for averting publicity to harmful chemical materials and pollutants:

Read the labels of all merchandise you buy to make sure they do no longer embody risky chemical materials.

The microbiome is the community of trillions of micro organism, viruses, fungi, and one-of-a-kind microorganisms that stay in and on our our bodies. These microorganisms play a important characteristic in our

health, by using helping us to digest meals, fight off infections, and regulate our immune gadget.

The microbiome is particular to all and sundry, and it is motivated by means of the use of the usage of a lot of of things, which include our genetics, our weight loss program, and our surroundings. The microbiome is continuously

changing, and it's miles essential to maintain a healthy microbiome on the way to live healthy.

There are some of techniques to preserve a healthful microbiome, collectively with consuming a wholesome diet, getting sufficient exercise, and reducing strain. Probiotics and prebiotics also can be

beneficial in supporting a wholesome microbiome.

The position of the microbiome in our health

The microbiome plays some of important roles in our health, together with:

Digestion: The microbiome allows us to digest food by using manner of breaking down complex carbohydrates and producing vitamins and particular vitamins.

Immune device: The microbiome allows to adjust our immune tool by using manner of producing antimicrobial materials and via education our immune machine to differentiate between harmless and

unstable micro organism.

Protection from ailment: The microbiome lets in to guard us from disease via manner of competing with dangerous micro organism for nutrients and with the useful aid of manufacturing antimicrobial materials.

Mental health: The microbiome also can play a position in highbrow fitness, with the resource of influencing our mood and behavior.

How to hold a healthy microbiome

There are numerous of things you could do to preserve a healthy microbiome, which consist of:

Eat a healthy healthy eating plan: A wholesome food regimen this is wealthy in culmination, vegetables, and complete grains can help to help a healthful microbiome.

Get sufficient exercising: Exercise can assist to promote the increase of beneficial bacteria within the microbiome.

Reduce pressure: Stress can negatively effect the microbiome, so it's far important to find techniques to manipulate strain for your existence.

Take probiotics and prebiotics: Probiotics and prebiotics are meals or dietary supplements that can assist to resource the increase of beneficial bacteria within the microbiome.[The Human Microbiome Project](

[The National Institutes of Health Microbiome Program]([The American Academy of Microbiology Microbiome Resource](How does the microbiome have an effect on our fitness?

The microbiome is the network of trillions of micro organism, viruses, and different microorganisms that stay in and on our bodies. These microbes play a critical function in our fitness by means of the use of

assisting us to digest food, combat off infections, and regulate our immune tool.

Here are a number of the strategies that the microbiome influences our fitness:

Digestion: The microbiome permits us to digest meals with the aid of breaking down complicated carbohydrates and generating enzymes that help us to absorb vitamins.

Immunity: The microbiome allows to modify our immune machine with the useful resource of producing molecules that fight off infections and with the useful useful resource of education our immune tool to distinguish among

unstable and innocent micro organism.

Allergies and hypersensitive reactions: The microbiome might also additionally

additionally play a characteristic in allergies and bronchial asthma by using influencing the development of our immune machine. Some studies have shown that humans with

allergic reactions and allergies have one-of-a-kind microbiomes than individuals who do now not have those situations.

Metabolism: The microbiome allows to modify our metabolism by using using producing molecules that assist us to break down and absorb vitamins. The microbiome also can play a function in

weight troubles and diabetes.

Mood and conduct: The microbiome also can have an effect on our mood and behavior by way of manner of the use of producing molecules that have interaction with our thoughts. Some studies have proven that people with depression and tension have one-of-a-kind microbiomes than folks who do no longer have those situations.

The microbiome is likewise involved in a number of chronic illnesses, which encompass weight issues, diabetes, and Crohn's sickness. By understanding how the microbiome impacts our fitness, we

can increase new remedies for those ailments and decorate the lives of thousands and thousands of people.

The microbiome is a powerful stress in our fitness, and through knowledge the manner it really works, we will learn how to beautify our health and nicely-being.

Here are some suggestions for improving your microbiome:

Eat a wholesome weight loss program that includes plenty of culmination, vegetables, and complete grains.

By following those pointers, you can help to beautify your microbiome and promote your normal fitness and properly-being.

The Future of the Microbiome

The microbiome is a abruptly evolving state of affairs of research, and there is but lots that we do not know about it. However, what we do recognize is that the microbiome performs a vital function in

our health, and with the aid of manner of facts the manner it really works, we are able to discover ways to beautify our health and nicely-being.

In the destiny, we're able to assume to see greater studies into the microbiome, and we're able to count on to see new treatments superior for a number of chronic illnesses. We also can count on to see new merchandise inside the marketplace that assist to assist a healthful microbiome.

The microbiome and persistent diseases

The microbiome is noted now to play a feature in a number of continual illnesses, along with weight troubles, diabetes, Crohn's sickness, and irritable bowel syndrome. This is because the

microbiome facilitates to adjust our immune device, our metabolism, and our digestion. When the microbiome is out of stability, it could contribute to the development of these persistent ailments.

In the future, we can anticipate to appearance new treatments developed for continual illnesses that focus on the microbiome. These treatments may additionally moreover moreover include using probiotics, prebiotics, or fecal microbiota transplantation (FMT).

Probiotics are stay microorganisms that might assist to enhance the stability of the microbiome. Prebiotics are non-digestible carbohydrates that feed the beneficial micro organism inside the

microbiome. FMT is a way in which fecal preserve in mind from a wholesome donor is transplanted into the recipient.

These remedies are however in the early degrees of development, but they show first-rate promise for the destiny of treating persistent illnesses.

The microbiome and the immune device

The microbiome plays a essential characteristic in our immune tool. The useful bacteria inside the microbiome assist to guard us from infection by way of manner of the use of producing antimicrobial substances

The microbiome furthermore performs a function in our metabolism. The beneficial micro organism inside the microbiome assist to digest meals, produce vitamins, and modify our blood sugar levels. When the

microbiome is out of balance, it can purpose weight benefit, obesity, and diabetes.

In the future, we are able to assume to look new remedies superior that focus on the microbiome to treat metabolic problems which consist of weight issues and diabetes. These remedies can also incorporate

the use of probiotics, prebiotics, or one-of-a-kind compounds that modulate the microbiome.

The microbiome and the destiny of medicine

The microbiome is a trendy frontier in medicine, and it's miles an interesting time to be studying it. By know-how how the microbiome works, we can discover ways to improve our health and

nicely-being, and we're able to create a more healthful destiny for ourselves and for generations to come back again.

Here are some of the methods that the microbiome is predicted to change the destiny of medicine:

New treatments for continual ailments. As we take a look at greater approximately the function of the microbiome in continual illnesses, we can be able to amplify new treatments that target the microbiome. These treatments may incorporate using probiotics, prebiotics, or FMT.

New recovery approaches for immune problems. The microbiome performs a crucial role in our immune system, and with the resource of knowledge how the microbiome works, we're able to be capable of increase new

treatment options to address immune problems collectively with allergic reactions, hypersensitive reactions, and autoimmune ailments.

New strategies to weight loss and weight problems. The microbiome performs a characteristic in our metabolism, and through the usage of information how the microbiome works, we can be able to extend new

techniques to weight loss and obesity.

New treatments for diabetes. The microbiome performs a position in our metabolismWhat is Gene Editing?

Gene enhancing is a form of genetic engineering that permits us to trade the

DNA of living organisms. This era has the capacity to revolutionize medicinal drug thru curing sicknesses,

treating genetic problems, or maybe improving our physical and intellectual abilities.

How does gene improving artwork?

Gene improving works through the use of quite some gadget to make specific adjustments to DNA. One not unusual gene improving tool is CRISPR-Cas9, which uses a protein known as Cas9 to reduce DNA

Chapter 6: Additional Assets

[The CRISPR Revolution: How Gene Editing Will Change the World](via

Jennifer Doudna and Samuel Sternberg

[Gene Editing: An Introduction](through the use of using the Nature Education group

[The Ethics of Gene Editing](by means of the National Human Genome Research InstituteHow Does Gene Editing Work?

Gene modifying is a effective generation that lets in scientists to trade the DNA of living organisms. This may be used to address illnesses, decorate crop yields, or create new organisms with favored dispositions.

CRISPR-Cas9

CRISPR-Cas9 is a gene modifying device that makes use of a protein known as Cas9 to lessen DNA at a specific place. CRISPR-

Cas9 works thru first identifying a quick piece of RNA that fits a

particular series of DNA. This RNA is then related to the Cas9 protein, which bureaucracy a complicated that binds to the DNA. Once the Cas9-RNA complex binds to the DNA, the Cas9 protein cuts the

DNA on the region in which the RNA fits the DNA series.

The CRISPR-Cas9 gadget may be used to edit genes in a number of organisms, which encompass bacteria, flowers, and animals. CRISPR-Cas9 has been used to cope with ailments which include sickle

mobile anemia and cystic fibrosis, and it has moreover been used to improve crop yields and create new organisms with preferred trends.

TALENs

TALENs are every different shape of gene modifying tool that makes use of a form of protein referred to as TALE to lessen DNA at a selected area. TALEs are proteins which can be made from a repeated series

of amino acids. Each repeat within the TALE protein binds to a selected base in DNA. This allows TALEs to bind to DNA in a selected order, which permits them to lessen DNA at a specific area.

TALENs can be used to edit genes in a whole lot of organisms, at the side of bacteria, plant life, and animals. TALENs have been used to deal with illnesses which includes sickle mobile anemia and cystic

fibrosis, and that they have additionally been used to beautify crop yields and create new organisms with favored tendencies.

Gene Editing Risks

Gene improving is a effective generation, but it additionally comes with a few risks. One risk is that gene enhancing may be used to create fashion style clothier toddlers or to alter people's genes in strategies that could have unintended effects. Another hazard is that gene improving can be used to create viruses or bacteria which may be proof in competition to antibiotics.

Despite the ones risks, gene improving is a promising technology that has the potential to revolutionize medicine and decorate human health. As scientists preserve to investigate extra about

gene improving, they may be able to develop techniques to apply this era effectively and correctly. Illnesses, address genetic troubles, or even beautify our physical and mental abilities.

Potential Benefits of Gene Editing

The capability blessings of gene enhancing are huge. This generation may be used to:

Cure illnesses. Gene enhancing might be used to goal and spoil genes that motive ailments which incorporates most cancers, cystic fibrosis, and sickle cell anemia. This have to bring about new and

more effective treatments for the ones diseases, or maybe treatments.

Treat genetic issues. Gene modifying may be used to correct genetic mutations that cause genetic troubles together with Huntington's sickness and muscular dystrophy. This must

reason improved first rate of life or even a therapy for the ones troubles.

Improve our bodily and intellectual competencies. Gene enhancing is probably used to beautify our bodily and intellectual capabilities. This should embody developing our energy, intelligence,

and reminiscence. It additionally may be used to treat situations on the facet of weight issues and intellectual infection.

Risks of Gene Editing

While gene modifying has the capability to revolutionize treatment and human fitness, it's far critical to keep in mind that this generation remains in its early ranges of improvement. There are a number of dangers associated with gene improving, which encompass:

Off-goal effects. Gene enhancing system can every so often edit genes that they are not purported to edit. This can purpose accidental element effects, collectively with genetic problems or maximum cancers.

Gene switch. Gene improving device can occasionally insert genes into the incorrect cells or into the incorrect place inside the genome. This can purpose unintentional side effects, together with

maximum cancers.

Gene escape. Gene edited cells can once in a while break out from the frame and spread to other people. This should purpose the spread of genetic problems or splendid sicknesses.

The Future of Gene Editing

The destiny of gene improving is unsure. There are a number of annoying situations that need to be conquer earlier than this generation can be used very well and successfully. However, the capability benefits of gene improving are so high-quality that it's miles simply nicely well worth pursuing this era but the dangers.

With cautious research and improvement, gene improving should eventually be used to treatment Gene improving is a effective new era with the functionality to revolutionize treatment and human health. However, it's miles essential to don't forget that this period continues to be in its

early tiers of improvement and that there are a number of dangers associated with it. It is essential to cautiously recollect the capability benefits and dangers of gene editing earlier than the usage of this

generation.

How CRISPR-Cas9 Works

CRISPR-Cas9 is a gene-enhancing device that permits scientists to make unique adjustments to DNA. It is a protein-guided RNA device. CRISPR-Cas9 works with the aid of first targeted on a specific gene with a guide RNA. The manual RNA binds to the DNA near the gene which you need to edit, and this recruits the Cas9 protein to the website on line. The Cas9 protein then cuts the DNA at a particular

area, which creates a break within the DNA. The cellular's natural DNA repair mechanisms then come into play, and they might each restore the DNA spoil or insert new DNA on the harm.

Components of CRISPR-Cas9

CRISPR-Cas9 is composed of maximum essential components: a manual RNA and a Cas9 protein.

The guide RNA is a quick piece of RNA that is complementary to a selected location of DNA. It courses the Cas9 protein to the appropriate place on the DNA.

The Cas9 protein is an enzyme that cuts DNA at a specific location. It is activated via manner of the guide RNA.

How CRISPR-Cas9 Works

The CRISPR-Cas9 machine works in three steps:

1. Target popularity. The guide RNA binds to the DNA near the gene which you need to edit. This recruits the Cas9 protein to the web page.

2. DNA reducing. The Cas9 protein cuts the DNA at a particular vicinity, which creates a harm inside the DNA.

3. DNA repair. The mobile's natural DNA repair mechanisms come into play, and they're able to every restore the DNA wreck or insert new DNA at the destroy.

Uses of CRISPR-Cas9 Biotechnology. CRISPR-Cas9 may be used to create new organisms with applicable traits. This must result in new crops which might be more evidence against pests and diseases, or new

biofuels that are more inexperienced to deliver.

Safety troubles

There are a few protection problems related to CRISPR-Cas9. For example, CRISPR-Cas9 need to doubtlessly be used to edit genes in a manner that might motive unintentional outcomes.

Additionally, CRISPR-Cas9 is probably used to create gene-edited organisms that could pose a hazard to human health or the environment.

CRISPR-Cas9 is a effective gene-editing device with a huge kind of functionality packages. However, there are also a few protection troubles associated with CRISPR-Cas9. It is critical to weigh the potential blessings of CRISPR-Cas9 towards the dangers earlier than the usage of this generation.

Applications of CRISPR-Cas9

CRISPR-Cas9 is a gene-enhancing device that has revolutionized the manner we observe and manage genes. It is a as an alternative new generation, but it has already had a high effect on many

fields, together with:

Studying gene function. CRISPR-Cas9 may be used to delete, insert, or replace genes in living cells. This lets in scientists to have a take a look at the characteristic of genes in extraordinary

detail. For instance, CRISPR-Cas9 has been used to find out genes which might be concerned in illnesses alongside aspect most cancers and cystic fibrosis.

Developing new remedies for sicknesses. CRISPR-Cas9 may be used to purpose and damage genes that purpose ailments. This need to cause new remedies for a extensive type of

ailments, inclusive of most cancers, sickle mobile anemia, and HIV.

Creating new plant life. CRISPR-Cas9 may be used to adjust vegetation to persuade them to more proof against pests, ailments, and environmental stresses. This must result in a more sustainable

food deliver.

Improving business organization methods. CRISPR-Cas9 can be used to regulate micro organism and distinct microorganisms to provide new chemical substances and materials. This should result in new strategies to

[CRISPR-Cas9: Applications in Agriculture](

[CRISPR-Cas9: Applications in Industrial Processes]([CRISPR-Cas9: Applications in Protecting the Environment](The Potential Benefits of Gene Editing

Gene improving is a all of sudden growing generation that has the functionality to revolutionize remedy and human health. By altering genes, gene modifying can be used to treatment sicknesses,

cope with genetic issues, or even decorate our physical and intellectual abilties.

Cure illnesses

Gene improving can be used to aim and ruin genes that purpose illnesses, which includes maximum cancers or sickle mobile anemia. For instance, a gene enhancing approach called CRISPR-Cas9 can be

used to reduce out a gene this is inflicting most cancers. This should stop the maximum cancers from growing and spreading.

Chapter 7: Treat Genetic Troubles

Gene editing also can be used to accurate genetic mutations that motive disorders, together with cystic fibrosis or Huntington's sickness. For instance, CRISPR-Cas9 can be used to

insert a wholesome duplicate of a gene right proper right into a cellular that has a mutation. This may want to allow the cell to deliver the protein that it needs, and the illness is probably dealt with.

Improve our bodily and mental abilties

Gene improving can also be used to beautify our physical and intellectual competencies, including our power, intelligence, or reminiscence. For example, CRISPR-Cas9 may be used to growth the

production of a protein this is involved in muscle growth. This may make us more potent. CRISPR-Cas9 may also be used to increase the form of synapses in our brains. This might also make us

smarter.

The capability benefits of gene modifying are massive, however it is vital to be privy to the functionality dangers as properly.

Off-goal outcomes

Gene modifying isn't always a sincerely perfect technology, and it is viable that it may through coincidence modify genes that we do now not intend to alter. This may also need to result in unintended facet effects,

Gene pressure is a era that might be used to unfold a preferred gene in the direction of a population. This is probably used to do away with diseases, but it is able to additionally be used to introduce unwanted trends right into a population.

Social and moral implications

Gene enhancing will growth some of social and ethical questions, which include who need to have get right of access to to this era, and the way it want for use. It is essential to cautiously endure in mind

the ones problems before gene enhancing is used on a huge scale.

Despite the dangers, the capability blessings of gene enhancing are so top notch that it's far definitely worth pursuing this period cautiously. With careful research and development, gene improving need to revolutionize medication and human health for the higher.

Here are some particular examples of the way gene improving may be used to deal with diseases and problems:

Cancer: Gene enhancing can be used to purpose and harm cancer cells. For example, CRISPR-Cas9 might be used to lessen out a gene this is using maximum cancers boom. This must

stop the cancer from developing and spreading.

Sickle cell anemia: Sickle mobile anemia is a genetic ailment that reasons purple blood cells to grow to be sickle-customary. This can purpose a number of fitness troubles, which embody pain,

anemia, and organ damage. Gene improving may be used to correct the mutation that reasons sickle cell anemia. This would possibly allow the frame to provide healthful red blood cells.

Cystic fibrosis: Cystic fibrosis is a genetic sickness that influences the lungs and digestive gadget. It is because of a mutation inside the CFTR gene. Gene editing can be used to insert a wholesome reproduction of the CFTR gene into cells. This should allow the cells to provide the protein that they want, and the illness could be treated.

Huntington's sickness: Huntington's ailment is a genetic sickness that motives modern thoughts damage. It is due to a mutation inside the HTT gene. Gene enhancing may be used

to correct the mutation that motives Huntington's sickness. This could prevent the sickness from progressing.

These are only some examples of the way gene improving is probably The Risks of Gene Editing

Gene improving is a effective new technology that has the potential to revolutionize treatment and agriculture. However, there also are some of risks related to gene modifying,

It is critical to cautiously undergo in mind the ones troubles in advance than gene enhancing is used on a massive scale.

Off-intention consequences

One of the maximum crucial risks of gene editing is that it could by way of accident alter genes that we do now not intend to regulate. This must reason unintentional issue outcomes, together with most cancers or one-of-a-kind fitness issues.

For instance, a take a look at posted inside the mag Nature in 2018 located that CRISPR-Cas9 gene editing must motive off-purpose outcomes in human cells. The observe located that CRISPR-Cas9

can also need to regulate genes that have been placed as lots as 100 base pairs away from the purpose gene. This should reason loads of accidental thing results, which consist of most cancers or different fitness troubles.

Another have a observe, published inside the mag Cell in 2019, observed that CRISPR-Cas9 gene enhancing also can reason off-target consequences in human embryos. The have a look at decided that CRISPR-Cas9

want to alter genes that have been positioned as heaps as one hundred,000 base pairs a long way from the intention gene. This may additionally need to bring about plenty of unintended aspect results, collectively with beginning defects or one-of-a-kind fitness troubles.

Gene pressure

Gene force is a technology that might be used to unfold a preferred gene during a populace. This might be used to put off ailments, along with malaria or HIV, or it can be used to introduce desirable trends into a populace, including resistance to pests or drought.

However, gene electricity furthermore has the potential to be used for malicious skills, in conjunction with introducing undesirable inclinations right into a population or developing splendid-weeds which is probably resistant

to herbicides.

Social and ethical implications

Gene enhancing will increase some of social and moral questions, which include who ought to have get proper of entry to to this generation, and how it want to be used.

Some people argue that gene enhancing must first-rate be used for restoration features, together with to deal with sicknesses or disabilities. Others argue that gene improving must additionally be used for enhancement purposes, which incorporates to improve athletic everyday ordinary performance or intelligence.Conclusion

Gene editing is a effective new generation with the functionality to revolutionize treatment and agriculture. However, there also are some of dangers related to gene enhancing,

consisting of off-intention outcomes, gene force, and social and ethical implications.

It is crucial to carefully don't forget the capacity advantages and dangers of gene enhancing earlier than this era is used on a large scale.

The Future of Gene Editing

Gene enhancing is a swiftly developing era that has the ability to revolutionize remedy. This technology permits scientists to alternate the DNA of an organism, that could

be used to remedy ailments, deal with genetic troubles, and even improve our physical and intellectual competencies.

The Benefits of Gene Editing

The functionality blessings of gene modifying are huge. This generation can be used to:

Cure illnesses. Gene enhancing will be used to intention and damage genes that cause ailments collectively with maximum cancers, cystic fibrosis, and sickle cellular anemia. This should bring about new and

more effective treatments for these illnesses, and will even cause treatment plans.

Treat genetic problems. Gene improving may be used to accurate genetic defects that motive genetic problems which encompass Down syndrome and muscular dystrophy. This ought to lead to

advanced notable of lifestyles for humans with those issues, and could even prevent them from being born inside the first location.

Improve our bodily and intellectual skills. Gene modifying might be used to beautify our physical and intellectual talents. This can also want to encompass making us stronger, quicker, smarter,

or extra proof in the direction of sickness. This can also want to have a exquisite impact on our lives, and could result in a more rich and healthy society.

The Risks of Gene Editing

While the functionality advantages of gene editing are tremendous, there are also some risks related to this era. These risks include:

The future of gene enhancing is unsure, but it has the functionality to revolutionize treatment. This era can be used to remedy ailments, cope with genetic issues, or even beautify our physical and intellectual talents. However, it is critical to be aware of the functionality risks of gene editing in advance than this era is used on a big scale.

Gene improving is a powerful generation that might have a incredible effect on the arena. It is crucial to cautiously do not forget the capability benefits and risks of this era before

it is used to exchange the human race.

Gene Therapy

Gene therapy is a shape of scientific remedy that entails introducing new genes into cells to treat or save you sicknesses. This may be executed via the usage of a virus to deliver the gene, or via using a non-viral transport technique. Gene treatment is a promising remedy for loads of diseases, which incorporates most cancers, cystic fibrosis, and sickle mobile anemia. However, gene remedy is

nevertheless in its early degrees of development, and there are risks associated with this generation. It is vital to talk over with a physician earlier than thinking about gene remedy.

How does gene remedy art work?

Gene remedy works by using the use of using introducing new genes into cells. These genes can then produce proteins that can each prevent or opposite the results of a disorder. For example, in the case of

most cancers, gene remedy may be used to introduce genes that code for proteins that inhibit the increase of maximum cancers cells.

What are the precise varieties of gene treatment?

There are principal styles of gene remedy:

Ex vivo gene treatment: In this shape of gene remedy, cells are removed from the frame, the genes are changed, after which the cells are lower back to the frame.

In vivo gene remedy: In this form of gene remedy, genes are brought right away into cells in the body.

What are the risks of gene therapy?

There are some of risks related to gene remedy, including:

Side effects: Gene treatment can motive factor consequences, together with infection, contamination, and toxicity.

Gene treatment has the capability to treat a extraordinary form of illnesses, which incorporates:

Cancer: Gene treatment may be used to aim most cancers cells and stop them from developing.

Cystic fibrosis: Gene remedy may be used to accurate the genetic infection that reasons cystic fibrosis.

Sickle cellular anemia: Gene treatment may be used to offer a lacking gene that is needed to produce hemoglobin, the protein that contains oxygen inside the blood.

What is the future of gene treatment?

Gene therapy remains in its early stages of improvement, however it has the capability to revolutionize the manner we address sicknesses. With similarly research, gene remedy must become a

secure and effective treatment for numerous illnesses.

References

[National Institutes of Health: Gene Therapy](

[Genetic Alliance: Gene Therapy](

[The American Society of Gene and Cell Therapy: Gene Therapy](CRISPR-Cas9 Gene Editing

CRISPR-Cas9 gene improving is a device that can be used to edit precise genes. This can be finished thru the use of CRISPR-Cas9 to reduce out a bit of DNA and update it with a brand new piece of DNA.

CRISPR-Cas9 gene modifying is a effective device that has the functionality to revolutionize the way we deal with ailments. However, CRISPR-Cas9 gene editing continues to be in its early degrees of development,

and there are risks related to this technology. It is critical to visit a medical scientific health practitioner earlier than considering CRISPR-Cas9 gene enhancing.

How CRISPR-Cas9 Gene Editing Works

CRISPR-Cas9 gene editing works via using a protein referred to as Cas9 to reduce DNA at a selected location. This place is determined with the resource of a quick piece of RNA, called a manual RNA (gRNA).

The gRNA binds to the DNA at the popular area, and the Cas9 protein then cuts the DNA.

Once the DNA is lessen, it can be repaired by using using the cell's natural DNA restore mechanisms. However, this restore manner can be exploited to introduce changes to the CRISPR-Cas9 gene improving has the potential to be used to address a massive type of illnesses. For instance, it can be used to:

Treat genetic sicknesses, which incorporates sickle cellular anemia and cystic fibrosis, via the use of correcting the mutations that purpose those ailments.

Develop new vaccines by way of focused on the genes of pathogens.

Create new flora which are evidence against pests and diseases.

Develop new biofuels and distinct renewable energy assets.

Risks of CRISPR-Cas9 Gene Editing

While CRISPR-Cas9 gene enhancing has the potential to revolutionize the way we cope with diseases, there are also risks related to this era. Some of the risks of CRISPR-Cas9

gene enhancing consist of:

Off-target effects: CRISPR-Cas9 can on occasion cut DNA at unintentional places.

This can bring about unintentional changes to the genome, that may likely have risky

effects.

Gene enhancing in germline cells: Germline cells are the cells that deliver rise to sperm and eggs. Editing germline cells can probably skip on genetic changes to future generations. This have to bring about new genetic illnesses or one-of-a-kind health problems.

Unintended consequences: CRISPR-Cas9 gene improving is a specifically new technology, and we do not however apprehend all the ability effects of using this era. It is

possible that CRISPR-Cas9 gene enhancing can also need to have accidental outcomes that we aren't privy to.

Chapter 8: Understanding the Immune System

As Bruce Lipton so aptly elements out, our bodies constantly have interaction with external threats the distinction among succumbing to a contamination or efficaciously fending it off lies within the kingdom of our immune system. To completely harness its energy, we first need to apprehend the intricacies of this complicated tool.

The Basics: How It Works

The immune device is much like a giant, difficult military, with severa specialized gadgets, each playing a selected function in our defense mechanism. These gadgets include cells, tissues, and organs, all taking element to protect us.

Imagine, if you'll, a grand citadel. The walls of this fort, comparable to our pores and skin and mucous membranes, act due to the truth the first line of safety, blocking off unwanted invaders. Beyond those partitions are the sentinels, or white blood cells, which continuously patrol and fight any breaches. These sentinels may be similarly classified into instructions, with some straight away attacking invaders at the same time as others produce antibodies, which could "hold in thoughts" and unexpectedly respond to previously encountered threats.

This functionality to "bear in mind" past invaders is what makes vaccines powerful. They introduce a innocent a part of a pandemic or micro organism, permitting our body to apprehend and remember it. So, if we come across the actual invader inside the destiny, our immune tool is primed to behave unexpectedly.

Factors that Weaken Immunity

In my years of workout, I've met human beings like James, a hardworking government in his 40s. James, constantly on the go with the flow, thrived on caffeine, slept slightly 5 hours a night, and determined solace in speedy meals. When he first walked into my health facility, he were combating a chronic bloodless for weeks. His tale offers a glimpse into the elements that might jeopardise our immunity.

1. Poor Nutrition: The fuel we provide our frame proper away influences its primary performance. Nutrient deficiencies, specially of vitamins C, D, and Zinc, can impair our immune characteristic.

2. Lack of Sleep: Our our bodies restore and rejuvenate at some point of sleep. Chronically reducing brief on rest compromises this recovery section, weakening our defenses.

three. Chronic Stress: Persistent pressure wreaks havoc on our immune gadget. It releases a hormone known as cortisol, which in extra, can suppress immune characteristic.

4. Excessive Alcohol and Tobacco: Both alcohol and tobacco can undermine our immune device. While moderate alcohol can be useful, immoderate consumption can keep away from the capability of white blood cells to fight viruses.

5. Sedentary Lifestyle: Regular physical interest enhances immune function. On the opposite, a sedentary manner of existence can purpose stagnation and reduced immunity.

Debunking Immune Myths

With an excellent amount of facts at our fingertips, it's clean to fall prey to myths. Let's debunk a number of the common misconceptions:

"Orange juice is an immune elixir": While oranges offer vitamins C, a important nutrient for immunity, completely counting on a tumbler of OJ during flu season isn't sufficient. Whole fruits, veggies, and a balanced weight-reduction plan are critical.

"I'm younger; I don't need to fear about my immunity": While it's proper that immunity can decline with age, younger people aren't invincible. Factors like strain, terrible eating regimen, and lack of sleep can weaken the immune gadget at any age.

"Taking greater nutrients manner better immunity": While vitamins are essential, extra isn't always higher. Excessive consumption, in particular of fats-soluble vitamins, may be risky. It's approximately stability and moderation.

Action Point:

Knowledge is empowerment. As you adventure via this ebook, use this foundational understanding of the immune device as your guide. This economic catastrophe underscores the significance of a holistic approach to fitness. Just as a sequence is simplest as strong as its weakest link, our immune gadget flourishes top notch while all contributing factors from food regimen to strain manipulate are addressed harmoniously.

Remember James, our overworked authorities. His story is a testomony that our each day choices play a pivotal function in figuring out our immunity's electricity. Every meal, each night time's rest, every workout consultation is a step within the course of constructing a resilient defense mechanism. Take charge of your immunity; it's a lifelong investment with immeasurable returns.

The Chiropractic Connection

This age-antique know-how from Hippocrates, the daddy of medication, is a testament to the undying precept of preventive fitness. In the arena of chiropractic, this preventive approach is paramount. What many might not recognize is the profound connection among chiropractic care and the body's immune reaction. Let's delve into this connection and discover its importance.

The Spine & Immunity Connection

The backbone is more than a structural column giving us form and form. It is the protecting casing for our spinal wire, a critical a part of our worried system. The hectic device, in turn, orchestrates and regulates all physical competencies, which includes the immune reaction.

Any misalignment or subluxation inside the spine can probably disrupt this verbal exchange channel. Think of it as a kink in a hosepipe, disrupting the drift of water. These misalignments can upward push up from different factors, be it posture, damage, or daily put on and tear. When spinal conversation faces disruption, the body may not respond as correctly to out of doors threats, compromising our immune function.

Regular Adjustments and Immune Response

Enter chiropractic changes. These are centered interventions to correct spinal misalignments, ensuring the gold ultra-modern go with the go together with the float of neural communications. Research has advised that chiropractic adjustments might result in a surge of immune-boosting cells, supporting in the frame's protection mechanism.

Maria, a schoolteacher in her 30s, changed into a shiny example of this. She first visited my exercise because of continual migraines. Along collectively with her debilitating complications, Maria frequently battled infections, from sinusitis to bronchitis. As her spinal fitness superior thru modifications, no longer handiest did her migraines reduce, but so did her frequency of infections. Over time, she transitioned from someone always below the weather to someone brimming with energy.

Case Studies from My Practice

Maria's story isn't an isolated incident. Over the years, I've visible severa instances wherein sufferers record more first-class immune feature alongside advanced spinal health.

Jake, a marathoner: After an uncongenial fall throughout a race, Jake suffered from persistent lower again pain. But, what alarmed him greater became a unexpected drop in his stamina and commonplace colds. As we embarked on a chiropractic treatment plan, no longer super did his over again ache alleviate, but he additionally located himself more resilient to infections.

Eleanor, an elderly retiree: Eleanor, stopping the aches and pains of age, started chiropractic care as a final inn for her sciatica. With everyday adjustments, Eleanor no longer only determined consolation from her sciatic pain but moreover located she should hold off the flu and colds an awful lot higher than numerous her peers. Her annual wintry weather bloodless became a hassle of the beyond.

Sam, a careworn govt: Consumed thru his table venture, Sam's posture suffered, fundamental to not unusual neck ache and stiffness. Alongside his bodily ache, Sam frequently found himself catching a few issue computer virus changed into circulating within the workplace. As he committed to ordinary chiropractic adjustments, not first-rate did his neck pain subside, however his days of sniffling and sneezing considerably reduced.

These recollections, from varying age agencies and backgrounds, all element to at least one reality: Our spinal fitness without delay influences our immune prowess.

Action Point:

In this journey toward fortified immunity, take into account about your spinal health. As showcased with the useful resource of manner of the memories and research, a well-aligned backbone may be a cornerstone to your immune defense technique. If you've in no manner considered chiropractic care, or probably relegated it honestly to ache control, it's time to re-have a look at.

Prioritise ordinary spinal check-u.S.And heed the advice of your chiropractor. Just as you wouldn't forget about about a weakened protection wall of a citadel, do now not overlook about about spinal misalignments that would potentially compromise your immune function.

Your spine is not simplest a shape; it's a conduit of lifestyles and power. Care for it, and it's going to take care of you in myriad techniques, immunity being a pinnacle instance. Embrace chiropractic as a pathway to holistic fitness and strong immunity.

Chapter 9: Nourishing Your Body Right

This profound assertion from the ancient Greek medical physician, Hippocrates, highlights a undying fact: The ingredients we eat play a pivotal function in our fitness and well-being. Now, in our quest for sturdy immunity, facts and utilizing the ideas of well nutrients becomes paramount. Let's embark in this culinary journey, uncovering the complicated courting amongst nutrients and immune fitness.

Basic Nutritional Principles

At its center, nutrients is ready stability. Our our our bodies require a myriad of vitamins, each serving a specific characteristic. Here are some foundational ideas to manual your nutritional selections:

1. Macronutrients Matter: Carbohydrates, proteins, and fat are the number one assets of energy for our our bodies. Each has a function to play. Carbohydrates are strength providers, proteins are critical for repair and boom, and fats – specially omega-3 and omega-6 fatty acids – assist mind characteristic and cell fitness.

2. Micronutrients Are Vital: Vitamins and minerals, despite the fact that required in smaller amounts, are important for numerous physical strategies. For example, Vitamin C aids collagen manufacturing and has antioxidant houses, whilst Zinc performs a feature in DNA synthesis and wound recovery.

3. Diversity Is Key: No single food can offer all the nutrients we want. Hence, a numerous eating regimen comprising numerous meals corporations guarantees we get a spectrum of nutrients.

4. Whole Over Processed: Opt for complete meals over processed ones. Processed foods frequently include components, preservatives, and hidden sugars, which provide little nutritional rate.

Everyday Foods with Immune-Boosting Benefits

During my consultations, I regularly encounter sufferers like Lisa, a hectic mother of 3. She as soon as confessed, "I understand I want to devour higher, but I certainly don't apprehend in which to start." Her sentiment resonates with many. While the marketplace is flooded with remarkable "superfoods", it's important to realize that regular substances, without troubles available, may be powerhouses of vitamins.

Garlic: A staple in plenty of kitchens, garlic consists of compounds like allicin, said for his or her immune-boosting homes.

Ginger: Often applied in teas or as a spice, ginger has anti-inflammatory and antioxidative houses.

Spinach: Rich in Vitamin C, antioxidants, and beta carotene, spinach complements our immune device's ability to fight infections.

Almonds: Packed with Vitamin E, essential for maintaining a wholesome immune device, just a handful may additionally want to make a distinction.

Yogurt: Probiotic-wealthy yogurt allows intestine fitness, a big contributor to immune function.

Remember Lisa? With minor adjustments and incorporating the ones normal elements into her circle of relatives's healthy eating plan, she noticed excellent modifications. Her youngsters were much less susceptible to seasonal colds, and she or he or he felt greater energised and colourful.

The Importance of Hydration

Water is the elixir of lifestyles. Every mobile, tissue, and organ requires water to feature successfully. From transporting nutrients to assisting digestion and flushing out pollution, water's roles in our body are manifold.

When we're thoroughly hydrated, our cells feature optimally, allowing our immune gadget to find and fight threats extra effectively. Furthermore, the mucous membranes, our body's first line of safety towards out of doors pathogens, stay moist and additional powerful at the same time as we're nicely-hydrated.

Action Point:

Your adventure to a nourished body and fortified immunity starts offevolved with aware alternatives. Start through way of evaluating your current weight loss plan. Where can you're making upgrades? Can you include more of the immune-boosting meals noted? Are you ingesting sufficient water day by day?

Remember, each meal is an opportunity to nourish and guide your frame. Like Lisa, small, ordinary modifications can bring about transformative consequences. Prioritise vitamins no longer in reality as a means to satiate starvation, but as a device to guide your body's defenses. Your immune system will thank you, and so will your common nicely-being.

5Adequate Sleep: The Underrated Immunity Booster

Thomas Dekker's terms resonate profoundly in these days's fast-paced global. While we frequently search for hard answers to reinforce our health, one of the maximum effective system lies proper in front humans: a very good night time's sleep. Let's find out the regularly-underestimated role of sleep in bolstering our immune defenses.

Understanding Sleep Cycles

Sleep isn't a monolithic kingdom of inactivity. Instead, it's a dynamic gadget comprising multiple cycles, every with its precise tendencies and capabilities.

1. NREM (Non-Rapid Eye Movement): This section is further divided into 3 levels:

Stage 1: A quick length of mild sleep, lasting a few minutes, sooner or later of which the coronary heart rate slows down and muscular tissues loosen up.

Stage 2: A deeper sleep characterized thru a further drop in body temperature and relaxation.

Stage 3: The inner most sleep degree, essential for physical recovery, increase, and strength replenishment.

2. REM (Rapid Eye Movement): Often associated with top notch dreams, REM sleep performs an important function in mind function, reminiscence consolidation, and temper regulation.

Throughout the night time time, we oscillate amongst those ranges, with each complete cycle lasting about 90 mins.

Tips for A Restful Night

Sophie, a freelance writer, as soon as approached me with persistent fatigue issues. She had attempted severa treatments, from dietary adjustments to meditation, with restricted fulfillment.

Upon closer inspection of her way of life, a big culprit emerged: erratic sleep styles. Here are some of the strategies we employed to beneficial resource Sophie in attaining more restful nights:

1. Consistency is Key: Stick to a ordinary sleep time table, even on weekends. This permits alter your frame's inner clock.

2. Create a Sleep-Inducing Environment: Ensure your mattress room is cool, dark, and quiet. Consider the use of earplugs, a watch colour, or a white-noise gadget if wanted.

three. Limit Screen Time: The blue mild emitted with the aid of telephones, computer systems, and TVs can intrude with melatonin manufacturing, a hormone answerable for sleep.

4. Watch Your Diet: Avoid heavy or big meals, caffeine, and alcohol earlier than

bedtime. These can disrupt sleep or cause ache due to indigestion.

5. Engage in Relaxing Activities: Consider studying, listening to calming song, or practising rest wearing sports activities in advance than mattress.

Sophie's transformation, as quickly as she started out engaging in consistent, restful sleep, became exquisite. Her fatigue faded, her cognitive talents sharpened, and he or she or he said feeling greater robust and plenty much less prone to common illnesses.

The Link between Sleep & Immune Function

Sleep isn't genuinely a length of relaxation for our brains and muscle businesses; it's a vital window for severa physiological strategies, immune function being one in each of them. Here's how they're intertwined:

1. Cytokine Production: During sleep, the body produces cytokines, a type of protein that goals infections and contamination. Lack of sleep can lessen the manufacturing of these protective cytokines.

2. Cellular Repair: The deep levels of sleep facilitate the restore and regeneration of cells, ensuring the advanced functioning of tissues and organs, together with those essential for immune protection.

three. Stress Hormone Regulation: Chronic sleep deprivation can cause stepped forward ranges of stress hormones like cortisol, which, ultimately, can suppress the immune device.

4. Efficient Immune Response: Studies advocate that right sufficient sleep can bolster the effectiveness of specialized immune cells referred to as T-cells. Conversely, sleep deprivation can lessen

the performance of these cells, making us more vulnerable to infections.

Action Point:

A restful night's sleep is not a luxurious; it's a non-negotiable for sturdy health and immunity. If you've been compromising on sleep, it's time to reset your priorities. As witnessed in Sophie's transformation, the ripple results of fine sleep move an prolonged way beyond feeling refreshed inside the morning.

In your quest for fortified immunity, permit sleep be your pleasant friend. Ensure you're giving your body the rest it deserves, allowing it to rejuvenate and prepare for something demanding conditions lie in advance. Embrace sleep not as a passive act but as an active funding in your fitness and well-being. Your immune device will thank you for it.

Chapter 10: The Role of Physical Activity

JFK's terms spotlight the holistic nature of physical health. Not most effective a gateway to a toned body, ordinary workout plays a foundational feature in intellectual properly-being, cognitive sharpness, and as we'll discover in this bankruptcy, bolstering immunity.

Exercise & Immunity: What Research Shows

Over the many years, a developing body of research has illuminated the beneficial relationship among normal bodily hobby and immune characteristic.

1. Improved Circulation: Exercise aids within the higher circulation of blood and lymphatic fluids. This way immune cells and antibodies flow into more swiftly, enhancing their capability to stumble upon and get rid of pathogens in advance.

2. Stress Regulation: Moderate exercising has been validated to lessen the discharge of strain hormones. Given that extended elevation of pressure hormones can suppress immune characteristic, normal physical interest acts as a buffer.

three. Enhanced Immunoglobulins: Studies recommend that people venture moderate ordinary workout have better tiers of immunoglobulins, which play a pivotal function in immune safety.

4. Reduced Inflammation: Regular physical interest can purpose a discount in persistent infection, that is related to severa fitness situations.

David, a 56-one year-antique accountant, serves as a testomony to those findings. Once main a sedentary way of life, David regularly decided himself struggling with minor infections. Upon incorporating regular bodily hobby into his recurring, not most effective did his health redecorate, however his susceptibility to infections additionally faded. He transformed from a ordinary on the nearby pharmacy to a person who barely remembered the ultimate time he had a cold.

Simple Workouts for Every Age & Ability

One of the misconceptions surrounding exercise is the perception that simplest immoderate, prolonged exercising sporting activities confer fitness blessings. This couldn't be similarly from the fact. Here are easy sporting events appropriate for various age organizations and abilties:

1. Seniors (Over 60): Gentle stretching bodily sports activities, tai chi, or short walks can show useful. Aquatic bodily sports, given their low effect, are also an remarkable desire.

2. Adults: From brisk walking, cycling, and swimming to domestic-based totally

absolutely resistance exercise workout routines using bands or frame weight, there are myriad alternatives. It's approximately locating an hobby you revel in, ensuring lengthy-term adherence.

3. Children: Traditional video games that contain walking, leaping, or perhaps dance-primarily based sports can make sure children are bodily energetic on the equal time as having a laugh.

four. Individuals with mobility challenges: Seated workout sports, which encompass top body actions or resistance bodily sports, may be useful. Additionally, physiotherapy can provide tailor-made workout sports.

Keeping Consistency: Motivation Tips

While know-how the importance of exercising is one trouble, preserving consistency can be a task. Here are a few pointers to stay stimulated:

1. Set Clear Goals: Whether it's undertaking a particular weight, strolling a high-quality distance, or genuinely feeling extra energetic, clean goals can act as a beacon.

2. Find an Exercise Buddy: Having a person to percent your fitness journey need to make workout workouts more fun and hold you accountable.

three. Mix It Up: Varying your exercise normal can save you monotony and maintain matters thrilling.

four. Celebrate Milestones: Achieved 10,000 steps each day for a month? Or swam a in addition lap? Celebrate these achievements, no matter how small.

5. Listen to Your Body: It's crucial to strike a balance. While it's appropriate to push yourself, overtraining may be destructive. Rest and healing are virtually as crucial.

Action Point:

Physical activity, as David's adventure showcases, is not quite a bargain aesthetics or athletic prowess. It's a crucial pillar of a strong immune tool. No depend your age or bodily scenario, there's an exercising regimen available tailored for you.

Begin nowadays. You don't must run a marathon or increase heavy weights. Start small, be regular, and steadily undertaking your self. Your immune device, like a silent cheerleader, will rally with strength, protecting you towards a number of the fitness traumatic conditions that come your manner.

Embrace physical interest, no longer as an occasional enterprise, but as a non-negotiable element of your each day existence. The rewards, each on the spot and extended-time period, may be properly nicely surely really worth the strive.

Mindfulness & Immunity

Dr. Dispenza's assertion encapsulates the profound hyperlink amongst our intellectual nicely-being and bodily health. While the location of mindfulness regularly gravitates towards discussions of intellectual peace and calmness, it performs a far less noted however further important feature in influencing our immune reaction. Let's dive deeper into the interplay amongst mindfulness and immunity.

Stress: The Silent Immune-Suppressor

Our our bodies are hardwired to reply to threats. Historically, those threats were at once and bodily a predator, for example. In reaction, the body would likely spark off the 'combat or flight' mode, liberating a surge of strain hormones. In in recent times's global, at the same time as predators are a rarity, our pressure responses are triggered regularly with the useful resource of each day stressful situations: tight closing dates, traffic jams, or financial concerns.

Chronic activation of this stress response can wreak havoc on our immune device. Here's how:

1. Inflammatory Response: Chronic stress has been connected to progressed tiers of infection in the body, doubtlessly principal to a group of diseases.

2. Suppression of Immune Cells: Prolonged exposure to strain hormones like cortisol can suppress the manufacturing and functioning of numerous immune cells, making us greater prone to infections.

three. Imbalance in Immune Response: Chronic pressure can purpose an imbalance in immune reaction, either making it overactive, as in the case of allergic reactions, or underactive, making us at risk of infections.

Linda, a devoted schoolteacher, changed into an illustrative case. She continuously felt beaten, juggling her expert commitments, dealing with her home, and searching after her growing old parents. As months rolled on, Linda determined herself often falling unwell. A communique about her intellectual properly-being found out the muse purpose: unmanaged pressure. Her relentless anxiety became not absolutely impacting her mind but suppressing her immune reaction.

Easy Meditation and Relaxation Techniques

The correct records? Mindfulness practices can act as effective antidotes to pressure, thereby not without delay bolstering our immunity. Here are a few smooth strategies:

1. Breathing Exercises: Focus to your breath. Inhale deeply for a rely of 4, maintain for four, and exhale for every different four. This approach can calm the thoughts almost proper now.

2. Guided Imagery: Close your eyes and don't forget a serene location possibly a beach or a meadow. Immerse yourself in the beauty and tranquility of this area, letting pass of all worries.

three. Progressive Muscle Relaxation: Starting out of your feet, hectic each muscle employer after which loosen up it, strolling your way up to your head.

4. Mindful Observation: Choose an object, perhaps a flower or perhaps your private hand. Observe it intently, noting its texture, color, and incredible data. This

exercise can anchor you to the existing second.

The Benefits of a Positive Mindset

A excessive nice thoughts-set doesn't suggest ignoring existence's disturbing situations or plastering a normal smile on one's face. Instead, it's approximately embracing a resilient and fine outlook. Here's the manner it impacts immunity:

1. Reduction in Stress Hormones: A first rate outlook has been associated with reduced stages of cortisol, thereby in a roundabout way helping immune feature.

2. Enhanced Antibody Production: Some research advise that an positive attitude can cause higher degrees of antibodies, imparting better safety within the path of pathogens.

3. Better Lifestyle Choices: Individuals with a effective attitude are more likely to have

interaction in health-selling behaviors like normal exercise, balanced nutrients, and good enough sleep, all of which in a roundabout manner increase immunity.

Action Point:

Mindfulness, as Linda decided, is extra than a buzzword. By embracing relaxation strategies and cultivating a pleasant attitude, she no longer best observed intellectual tranquility however additionally fortified her immune defenses.

Take a 2d every day to engage in mindfulness. Whether it's a quick meditation session, focused respiratory, or genuinely immersing your self in the beauty of nature, those practices can reset your pressure ranges.

Remember, a resilient mind fosters a resilient body. Prioritise your intellectual properly-being, and your immune device will genuinely observe in form, imparting you robust protection in opposition to the myriad annoying conditions of the out of doors worldwide.

The Chill Factor: Weighing Cold Water Swimming and Ice Baths

Wim Hof, seemed globally because the "Iceman," is famend for his advocacy of bloodless exposure as a manner to liberate human capability. He has drawn interest to practices like bloodless water swimming and ice baths, praising their myriad health benefits. But like each modality, they arrive with their professionals and cons. Let's dive deep into the chilling world of cold cures and apprehend their implications.

From The Lakes of Cumbria: An Illustrative Dive

In the serene lakes of Cumbria, Anna, a documentary filmmaker, met Eric, a seasoned bloodless-water swimmer. Erik, in his overdue 50s, swam each day, even in the frigid wintry weather months. Anna, to start with traumatic, decided to movie or even experience the bloodless plunge herself. Her venture into the icy waters and next immersion in an ice tub in some unspecified time inside the future of her stay have become transformative, however it additionally shed slight on the stark professionals and cons of such practices.

The Pros:

1. Boosted Immune Response: Regular cold publicity can enhance the immune device. Studies endorse that cold water swimmers display an growth in white blood cellular rely.

2. Improved Circulation: Cold water immersion forces the frame to streamline blood drift, improving go with the flow.

This can useful useful resource in muscle healing and reduce contamination.

3. Mental Fortitude: Just as Eric emphasised to Anna, pushing oneself to enter bloodless water or take an ice bathtub can build intellectual resilience, focus, and reduce signs of hysteria and melancholy.

four. Thermogenic Benefits: Exposure to cold can boom metabolism because the frame works to maintain its center temperature, potentially assisting in weight manipulate.

The Cons:

1. Initial Shock: The body's first reaction to bloodless is a wonder, which could spike blood stress and coronary coronary coronary heart rate. This might be destructive for people with cardiovascular troubles.

2. Hypothermia Risk: Extended exposure, particularly in quite cold situations, can result in hypothermia, a immoderate and doubtlessly deadly situation.

three. Muscle Numbness: Anna's preliminary plunge left her feeling numb and tingly, a common reaction. This can every so often bring about impaired coordination and capability damage.

four. Not for Everyone: While Eric ought to swim every day within the bloodless lakes, such practices might not suit all people, specifically those with excellent scientific conditions.

Action Point:

Anna's transformative journey with cold water swimming and ice baths come to be -fold. While she professional greater appropriate recognition, better sleep, or even decreased soreness from her hikes, she furthermore realised the importance of respecting her body's limits.

Your movement factor is to method cold water swimming and ice baths with each interest and warning. If intrigued, start frequently, in all likelihood with cooler showers. Always make certain protection, and if considering greater severe bloodless exposures, consult a scientific expert. Remember, at the equal time as the bloodless can definitely be an "sincere teacher," as Wim Hof says, it's essential to be a diligent student, taking note of and respecting your body's responses.

Chapter 11: Nature's Gift Sunshine and Fresh Air

Fitzgerald incredibly captures the rejuvenating spirit of nature. The solar, with its golden rays, doesn't simply brighten our environment however performs a pivotal role in our health, especially in phrases of our immune device. This financial ruin shines a mild on the simple hyperlink among nature's services—sunshine and glowing air—and our nicely-being.

Vitamin D: The Sunshine Vitamin

Our pores and skin's publicity to daylight triggers the synthesis of Vitamin D, frequently dubbed the 'Sunshine Vitamin.' Despite its name, Vitamin D is more than only a nutrition; it's a seasoned-hormone answerable for severa techniques within the frame.

1. Bone Health: Vitamin D is paramount in calcium absorption inside the gut, ensuring sturdy and healthful bones.

2. Mood Regulation: Deficiency in Vitamin D has been associated with temper problems, such as melancholy.

three. Immune Function: Vitamin D is critical for the right functioning of T-cells, which may be critical additives of the immune tool.

Emma, a contract writer, frequently discovered herself cooped up interior, engrossed in her work. Over time, she placed a decline in her energy ranges, common temper swings, and a propensity to fall sick. A recurring checkup unveiled a wonderful Vitamin D deficiency. It changed into clean: her indoor way of existence modified into depriving her of the multifaceted advantages of the sunshine diet.

Importance of Regular Outdoor Activities

Nature has a holistic effect on our well-being. Sunshine performs its element thru Vitamin D synthesis, however the sheer act of being outside gives severa high-quality benefits:

1. Improved Air Quality: Indoor air can frequently be extra polluted than outdoor air because of dirt mites, mildew, and different contaminants. Fresh air can rejuvenate and detoxify the frame.

2. Mental Well-being: Exposure to nature has been verified to reduce signs of anxiety, melancholy, and pressure.

three. Enhanced Immunity: Regular publicity to nature can decorate our immune feature. Phytoncides, obviously produced by means of the usage of vegetation, had been examined to enhance our white blood mobile interest.

Practical Ways to Incorporate Nature into Your Routine

While the advantages of nature are manifold, town life frequently limit our exposure. However, with some intentional strive, it's feasible to mix more of nature into our every day lives:

1. Morning Ritual: Begin your day with a brief stroll, jog, or perhaps some stretching bodily video games in a close-by park or lawn.

2. Lunch Breaks: If you're on foot, use part of your lunch destroy to take a short stroll out of doors. This now not fine gives publicity to daylight hours however additionally gives a intellectual destroy.

3. Indoor Plants: Bring nature to you. Indoor flowers can purify the air and raise your mood.

4. Weekend Activities: Dedicate weekends to outdoor sports activities activities—be it hiking, picnicking, or in reality analyzing a ebook in a serene environment.

five. Natural Light: Ensure your living and workspace has adequate herbal mild. Open home windows and curtains to permit the sunlight flood in.

Action Point:

Emma's journey serves as a effective reminder. Nature isn't truly a polished luxurious—it's a essential necessity for our holistic nicely-being. Following her prognosis, Emma made a aware effort to step out of doors each day, be it for artwork, leisure, or workout. The transformation grow to be palpable. Her strength degrees soared, her mood stabilised, and her immunity fortified.

Take a leaf out of Emma's ebook. Make it a every day goal to step outside, soak in a few daylight, and breathe in the freshness of nature. The sunshine and the rustle of leaves aren't simply sensory delights; they may be nature's elixir, promising a robust immune device and an invigorated spirit.

Every ray of daylight and every breath of easy air is a step inside the course of higher health. Embrace nature's present, and watch it paintings its wonders in your frame and soul.

Limiting Toxins in Your Environment

Lady Bird Johnson's phrases echo the obvious fact: the surroundings is our shared location. But, these days, our environment has come to be inundated with a myriad of pollutants. These invisible adversaries, often a made of our modern-day way of life, can inadvertently weaken our immune defenses. By recognizing and limiting them, we're able to reclaim our surroundings and beef up our health.

Everyday Toxins & Their Effects on Immunity

Every day, without us even identifying, we're uncovered to a mess of pollution. They lurk in our homes, places of work, or maybe the meals we eat:

1. Household Cleaners: Many industrial cleaners incorporate chemical substances which could purpose respiratory issues and skin irritations. They also can have prolonged-term effects on our hormonal and immune structures.

2. Pesticides: Residues from pesticides on our fruits and veggies can disrupt our endocrine device and dampen our immunity.

three. Air Pollutants: Emissions from motors, factories, and even some circle of relatives home system release pollutants that, whilst inhaled, can beat back lung function and obstruct the immune response.

4. Cosmetics & Personal Care Products: Parabens, phthalates, and sulfates, normally determined in lots of private care products, can be absorbed into our bodies, inflicting hormonal imbalances and lowering immune characteristic.

James, a metropolis-residing authorities, have emerge as in the top of his lifestyles. But he continuously battled fatigue, commonplace colds, and unexplained hypersensitive reactions. Investigating deeper, he realised his upscale urban lifestyle exposed him to a cocktail of pollution every day. From the air freshener in his rental to the pesticide-weighted down end result in his basket, pollution have been everywhere.

Clean Living: Simple Changes, Big Impact

While the list of pollution might also moreover appear daunting, some aware adjustments can substantially lessen our publicity:

1. Opt for Organic: Whenever possible, pick out out out natural produce. This guarantees that your food is unfastened from dangerous insecticides and chemical materials.

2. Ventilate: Ensure your dwelling areas are nicely-ventilated. This easy step can reduce indoor pollution notably.

3. Limit Plastic Usage: Plastics, especially at the equal time as heated, can release chemical substances. Use glass or chrome steel for garage and avoid microwaving meals in plastic bins.

4. Choose Natural Cosmetics: Opt for cosmetics and private care products which can be loose from risky chemical substances. Always have a look at labels

and be knowledgeable about what you're using for your pores and pores and skin.

Natural Cleaners & Products Recommendations

Making the switch to herbal products is not just about looking for one-of-a-type gadgets—it's approximately adopting a latest, toxin-loose way of life:

1. Vinegar & Baking Soda: This mixture is a powerhouse cleaner. It can clean surfaces, unclog drains, or even act as a material softener.

2. Essential Oils: Oils like tea tree, lavender, and lemon no longer only have cleaning residences but furthermore depart a nice aroma.

three. Castile Soap: An all-natural, biodegradable cleaning cleansing cleaning soap that may be used for the entirety—from dishwashing to frame wash.

four. Recommendation: Brands like Mrs. Meyer's, Seventh Generation, and Dr. Bronner's are stated for their inexperienced, herbal merchandise. They offer some of cleaning stores, laundry detergents, and private care merchandise with out the dangerous pollution.

Action Point:

James's tale changed into a turning point. He transitioned to herbal cleaners, swapped out his everyday prevent result for herbal alternatives, and scrutinised his personal care merchandise. The consequences had been glaring. His electricity returned, and he determined a awesome drop in his commonplace illnesses.

Take a cue from James. Begin via evaluating your environment. The pollution might be silent, but their effects are loud and clean. By making intentional options, you could limit the ones pollutants and provide a greater healthful surroundings for yourself and your loved ones.

Remember, the healthiest model of yourself isn't only a fabricated from what you eat, however additionally the surroundings you inhabit. Prioritise smooth residing and watch as your immune device flourishes in a cleanser, toxin-loose surroundings.

Community & Connection: Social Wellness

Montaigne's mirrored image on self-know-how and belonging underlines the profound importance of our connection to others and the wider community. Our social bonds aren't definitely assets of satisfaction and companionship—they play a critical role in our average nicely-being and, in particular, our immunity.

The Science of Social Bonds & Immunity

Interpersonal relationships have an impact on our health in severa, often surprising, strategies:

1. Stress Reduction: Positive social interactions can lower ranges of cortisol, the stress hormone. Chronic pressure is idea to suppress the immune system.

2. Emotional Support: Friends and circle of relatives act as buffers for the duration of tough times, imparting emotional assist which could, in turn, improve our physical fitness.

three. Healthier Habits: Being a part of a community or a close-knit agency often promotes extra healthful manner of existence choices, from workout to dietary behavior.

Sophia, a committed profession lady, often found solace in her paintings, however her non-public connections dwindled through the years. A fitness scare made her recognize that, even as she had expert achievements, she lacked a help device. This loneliness wasn't definitely an emotional challenge—it have become affecting her fitness.

Cultivating Meaningful Relationships

Nurturing relationships calls for intention and strive. Yet, the rewards, every emotional and physiological, are clearly worth the funding:

1. Active Participation: Engage in network activities, be it nearby workshops, organization health education, or network activities.

2. Open Communication: Foster open communicate with friends and circle of relatives. It permits in building be given as authentic with and information.

3. Lend a Hand: Volunteering no longer handiest strengthens network bonds but

has been verified to reinforce person nicely-being.

Staying Connected in a Digital World

The COVID-19 pandemic and the following lockdowns threw the arena right into a paradoxical scenario. On one hand, technology allowed us to stay connected, but on the alternative, bodily isolation became the norm. This contradiction had multifaceted implications:

1. Digital Fatigue: The over-reliance on virtual structures induced a phenomenon known as 'Zoom fatigue,' marked via exhaustion from excessive show show screen time.

2. Heightened Loneliness: Despite digital connections, the absence of physical interaction accentuated emotions of loneliness for hundreds.

three. Immune Impact: As referred to earlier, social bonds effect immunity. The isolation and stress from the lockdowns ought to very well have weakened immune defenses, including every other layer of vulnerability in the course of an already difficult time.

Action Point:

Sophia's epiphany changed into transformative. She actively sought out network engagements, reconnected with vintage friends, or even embraced the virtual global's nice factors to preserve connections. Over time, her fitness progressed, and he or she felt greater rooted in her community.

Take a 2nd to reflect in your connections. In a global teeming with virtual interactions, prioritise actual, heartfelt connections. While digital structures are gear of comfort, make certain they don't update the irreplaceable warm temperature of face-to-face interactions.

Let's studies from the annoying conditions posed with the useful resource of the pandemic: While we might be bodily apart, we want to find strategies to stay emotionally and socially related for our holistic well-being. Commit to fostering significant relationships, and witness the profound impact in your immunity and primary fitness.

Chapter 12: Steering Clear of Over-The-Counter Pitfalls

Paracelsus reminds us of the difficult dance between remedy, health, and our our bodies. While over the counter (OTC) pills offer quick comfort and luxury, it's important to be aware of their implications on our immune device and ordinary health. In this financial ruin, we will delve into the not unusual OTC drug remedies that would affect immunity, the vicinity of herbal alternatives, and the importance of being an informed purchaser.

Common Medications that Might Affect Immunity

The neighborhood pharmacy cabinets are blanketed with an array of OTC tablets, promising consolation from severa ailments. However, hundreds of these would possibly likely inadvertently compromise our immune reaction:

1. NSAIDs (Non-Steroidal Anti-Inflammatory Drugs): While they correctly combat contamination and ache, extended use can effect the immune device's ability to function optimally.

2. Decongestants: Useful for clearing a stuffy nostril, those can suppress additives of the immune reaction, making us extra prone to secondary infections.

3. Antibiotics: While now not constantly to be had over-the-counter in all global locations, their misuse or overuse can harm the stableness of accurate bacteria in our our bodies, essential for a robust immune tool.

Sarah, a marathon runner, relied closely on NSAIDs for pain treatment at some stage in her education. Over time, she placed herself falling sick regularly. It come to be complex—a person as in shape as her shouldn't be so susceptible to infection. A consultation decided out her ordinary NSAID use because of the reality the functionality culprit, affecting her immune defenses.

Natural Alternatives & When to Consider Them

Nature gives a plethora of remedies that may be effective without compromising immunity:

1. Turmeric & Ginger: Both very very own anti inflammatory houses, making them herbal alternatives to NSAIDs.

2. Echinacea: Known to enhance the immune gadget, it could be taken at the onset of bloodless signs and signs.

3. Probiotics: Maintaining gut fitness is vital for immunity. Natural probiotics like yogurt or fermented meals can be useful.

However, it's crucial to searching for advice from a healthcare professional in advance than making any giant adjustments to remedy or adopting herbal remedies. They can guide on dosages, interactions, and ability facet results.

Reading Labels & Being Informed

An empowered client is an knowledgeable one. Here are a few tips:

1. Active Ingredients: Always test the primary substances. This will assist in averting capacity drug interactions, in particular if you're already on one of a kind medicinal pills.

2. Side Effects: All drugs may additionally have issue consequences. Being aware can help in spotting symptoms early must they upward thrust up.

three. Dosage: Follow encouraged doses diligently. More doesn't continuously suggest higher or faster consolation.

four. Expiration Dates: Expired drug treatments may be a great deal less powerful and, in some instances, volatile.

Action Point:

Sarah's revelation changed her approach to pain manipulate. Instead of automatically achieving for NSAIDs, she started incorporating herbal anti-inflammatories into her diet plan and consulted her medical doctor approximately opportunity pain manage techniques. Her fitness superior, and she or he or he have become better organized to deal with the wishes of her schooling.

Your motion thing? Next time you're about to pick out out up a remedy, pause. Read the label very well, be informed about its results, and keep in mind if there's a natural alternative truely nicely well worth exploring. Always prioritise prolonged-time period nicely-being over short-term treatment.

Remember, at the equal time as drugs provide remedies, proper fitness is a stability of attention, knowledgeable options, and proactive care. Equip your self with records, and make alternatives that bolster, now not prevent, your body's natural defenses.

Regular Check-u.S.A. Of americaand Preventative Measures

Gandhi's words resonate deeply while we keep in mind our fitness. Serving our our bodies manner statistics them, nurturing them, and being proactive about our well-being. Regular take a look at-americaand preventative measures offer notion into our health, permitting us to act rapidly and accurately. In this chapter, we can apprehend the importance of information our essential health metrics, the placement of ordinary exams, and the wider image of preventative care.

Knowing Your Numbers: Basic Health Metrics

At the middle of expertise our fitness are positive critical metrics:

1. Blood Pressure: A critical indicator of cardiovascular fitness. Regular monitoring can offer early warnings for situations like immoderate blood stress.

2. Blood Sugar Levels: Helps in monitoring the body's potential to metabolise glucose. It's crucial for diagnosing and coping with diabetes.

3. Body Mass Index (BMI): While not a definitive measure of fitness, it may provide a latest information of weight in phrases of top.

James, a tech entrepreneur in his early 40s, taken into consideration himself pretty healthy. However, a ordinary check-up painted a completely unique image. Elevated blood pressure and blood sugar ranges were silent signs of lurking health problems. He realised that he couldn't absolutely rely on outside appearances or perceived well-being.

The Importance of Routine Medical and Chiropractic Exams

While we often are searching for medical interest at the same time as we're ill, normal tests play a pivotal characteristic:

1. Early Detection: Regular screenings can find ability fitness issues in advance than they grow to be immoderate. This early intervention may want to make treatments greater powerful.

www.ingramcontent.com/pod-product-compliance
Lightning Source LLC
Chambersburg PA
CBHW070554010526
44118CB00012B/1317